CHOCOLATE
its sexual power—with recipes

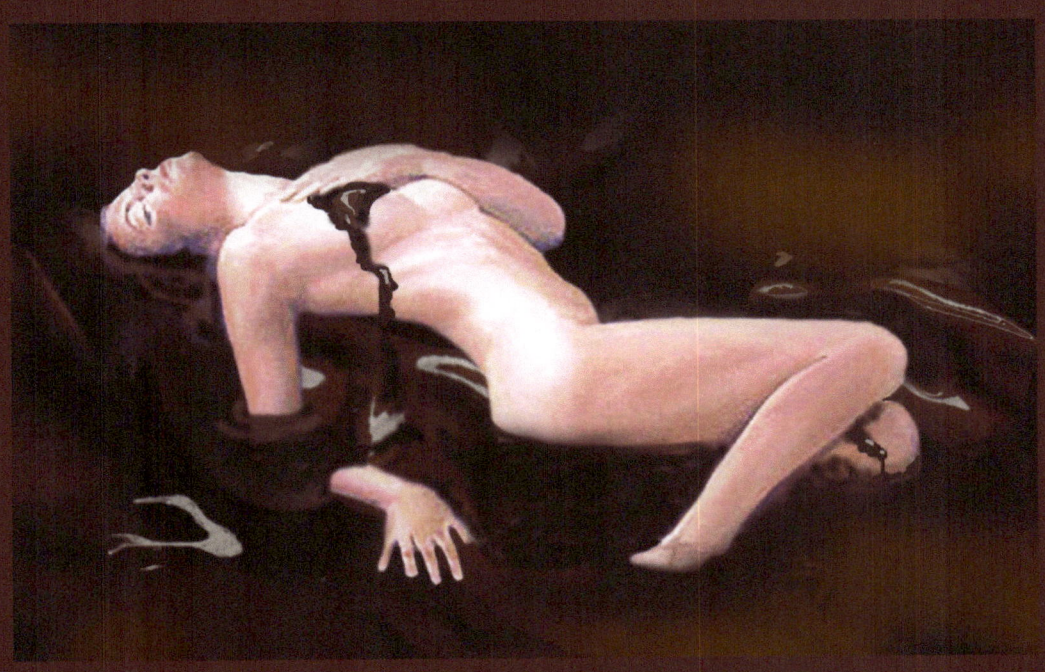

Louis E.V. Nevaer

Copyright © 2013 by Hispanic Economics, Inc.

Manufactured in the United States of America. All rights reserved. No part of this book may be reproduced in any form or by any means, electronic or mechanical, including photocopying, recording, or by information storage and retrieval systems—except by a reviewer who may quote brief passages in a review to be printed in a magazine, newspaper or on the Internet—without permission in writing from the publisher. This book is presented solely for educational and entertainment purposes. All the opinions expressed are those of the author and do not reflect those of Hispanic Economics, Inc., its employees or clients. Although the author and publisher have made every effort to ensure that the information in this book was correct at press time, the author and publisher do not assume and hereby disclaim any liability to any party for any loss, damage, or disruption caused by errors or omissions, whether such errors or omissions result from negligence, accident, or any other cause.

Medical disclaimer: This discussion presented in this book is not intended as a substitute for the medical advice of physicians. The reader should regularly consult a doctor in matters relating to his or her health and particularly with respect to any symptoms that may require diagnosis or medical attention. Ask your doctor if your heart is health enough for sexual activity. Ask your doctor if eating 30 to 40 grams (1 to 2 ounces) of 100 percent criollo dark chocolate is appropriate for you.

First printing 2013. Publication date: August 2013

ATTENTION CORPORATIONS, UNIVERSITIES, COLLEGES, AND PROFESSIONAL AND CHARITABLE ORGANIZATIONS: Quantity discounts are available on bulk purchases of this book for educational and gift purposes, or as premiums in fundraising efforts. Inquiries should be sent to info@hispaniceconomics.com.

Hispanic Economics, Inc.
P.O. Box 140681
Coral Gables, FL 33114-0681
info@hispaniceconomics.com
HispanicEconomics.com

ISBN 978-1-939879-03-5

All photographs provided by the author, except for the following:

"Binding My Muse," on page 22 and back cover, appears courtesy of the artist, Carolyn Weltman: 150 East 37 Street, #10-E, New York, NY 10016, www.carolynweltman.com. Facebook: https://www.facebook.com/carolyn.weltman.art

Illustration for "The Invention of Maize," on page 34, by Nicolle Rager Fuller, courtesy of the National Science Foundation.

The photograph for "Conflict Cacao," page 36, appears courtesy of the photographer U Roberto (Robin) Romano, Romano Film & Photography, Inc., P.O. Box 168, Mohegan Lake, NY 10547. Telephone: 917-669-4421. www.urobertoromano.com

Cover and Interior Design by John Clifton, john@johnclifton.net

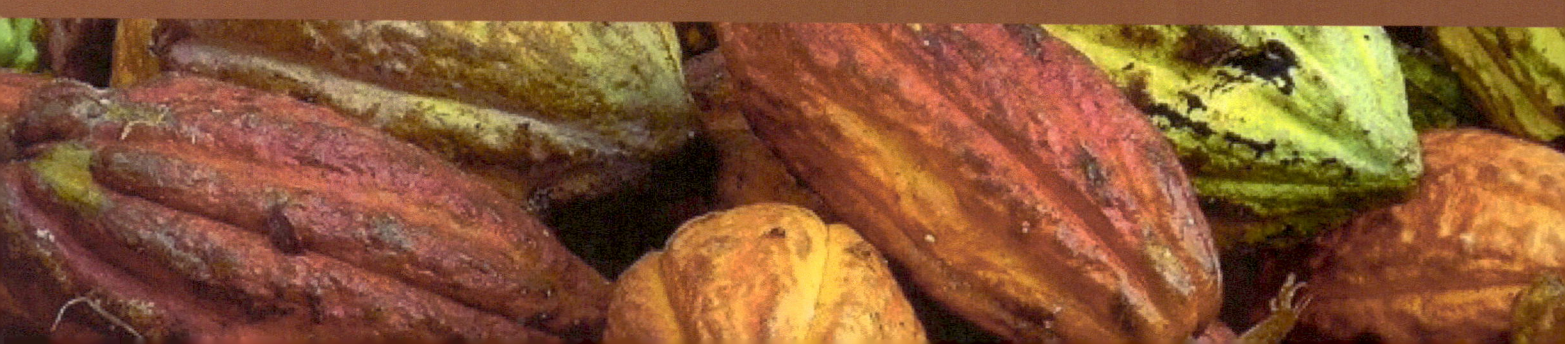

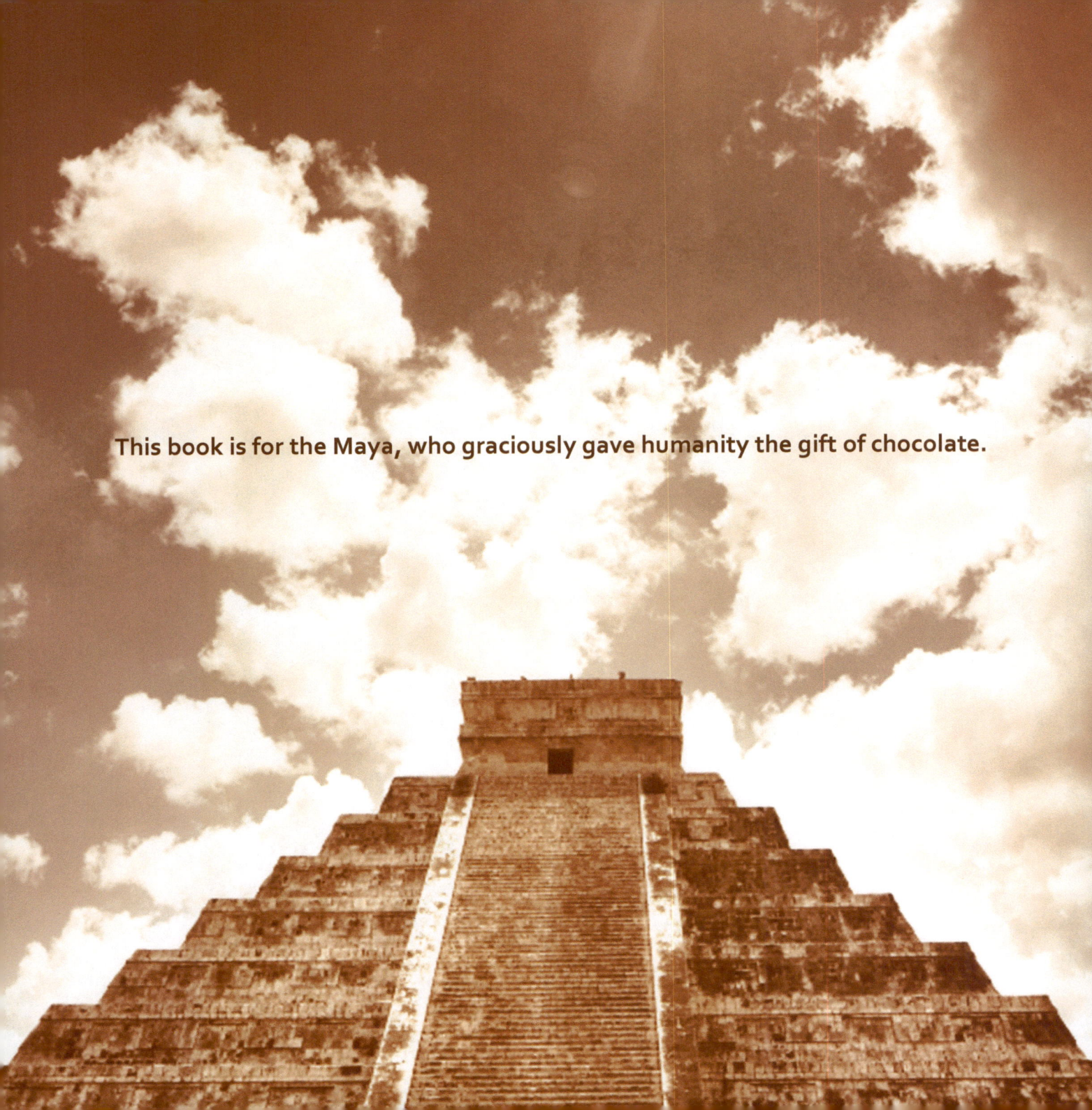

This book is for the Maya, who graciously gave humanity the gift of chocolate.

about the author

Louis E.V. Nevaer is a leading authority on the three great flavors of southern Mexico: mezcal, chocolate, and coffee. He divides his time between New York and Mexico, with no regrets.

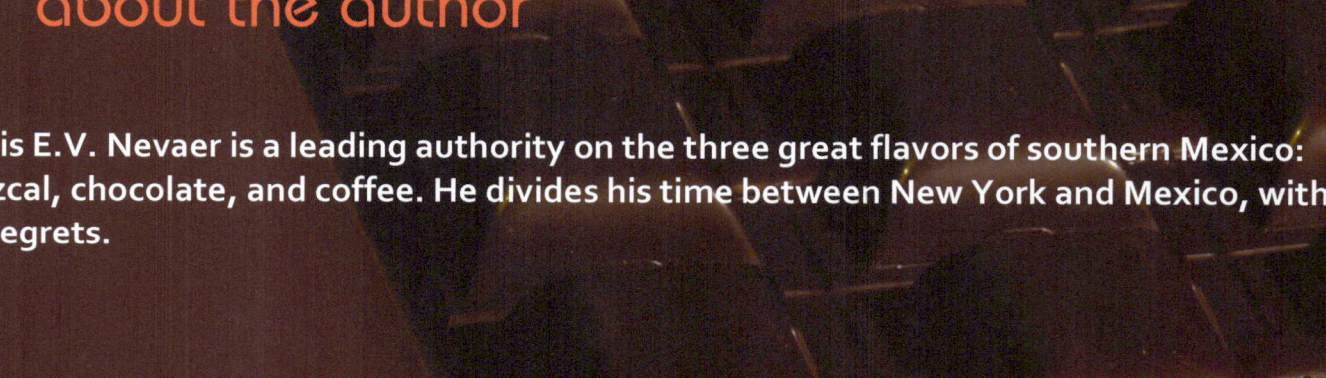

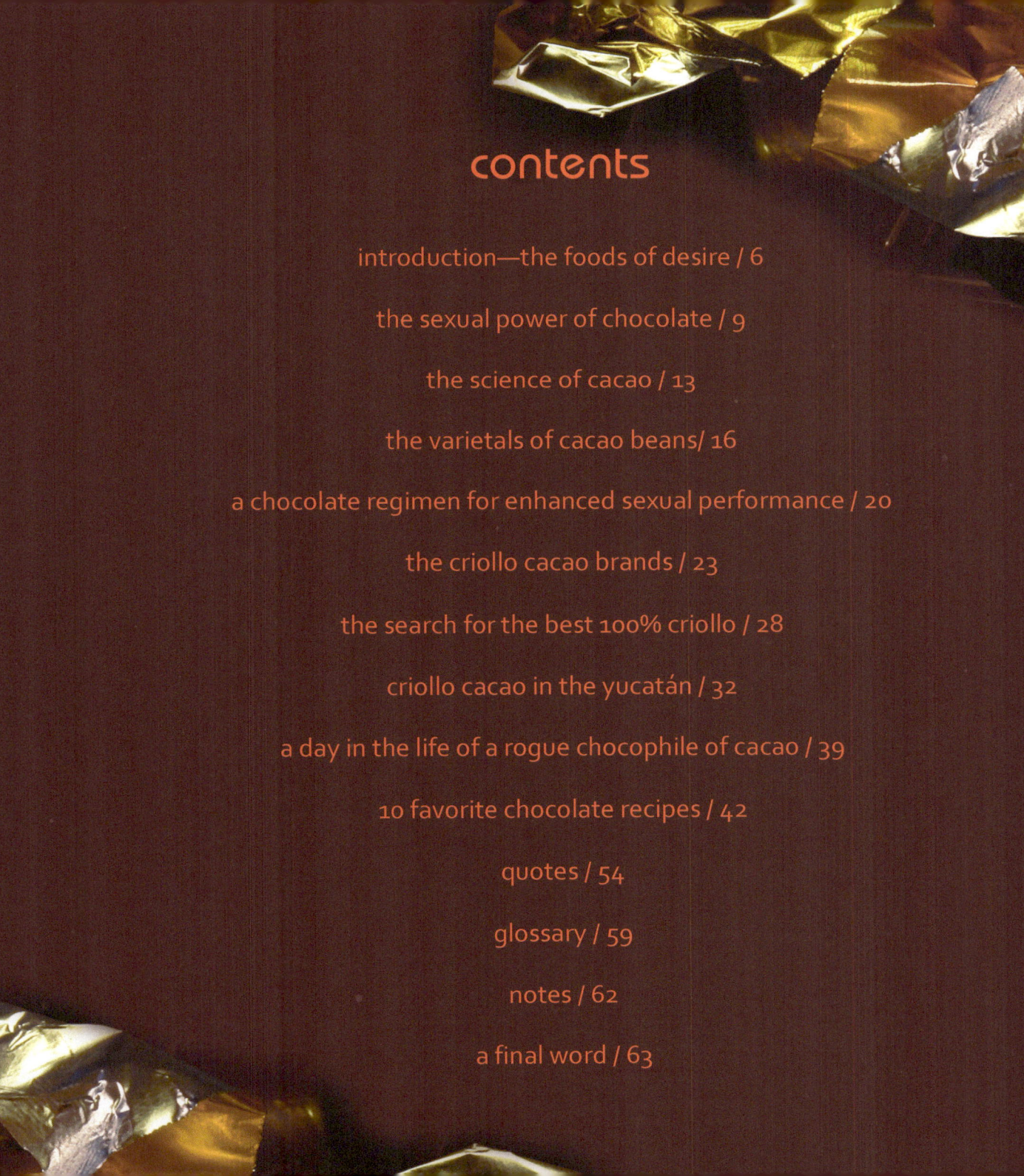

contents

introduction—the foods of desire / 6

the sexual power of chocolate / 9

the science of cacao / 13

the varietals of cacao beans / 16

a chocolate regimen for enhanced sexual performance / 20

the criollo cacao brands / 23

the search for the best 100% criollo / 28

criollo cacao in the yucatán / 32

a day in the life of a rogue chocophile of cacao / 39

10 favorite chocolate recipes / 42

quotes / 54

glossary / 59

notes / 62

a final word / 63

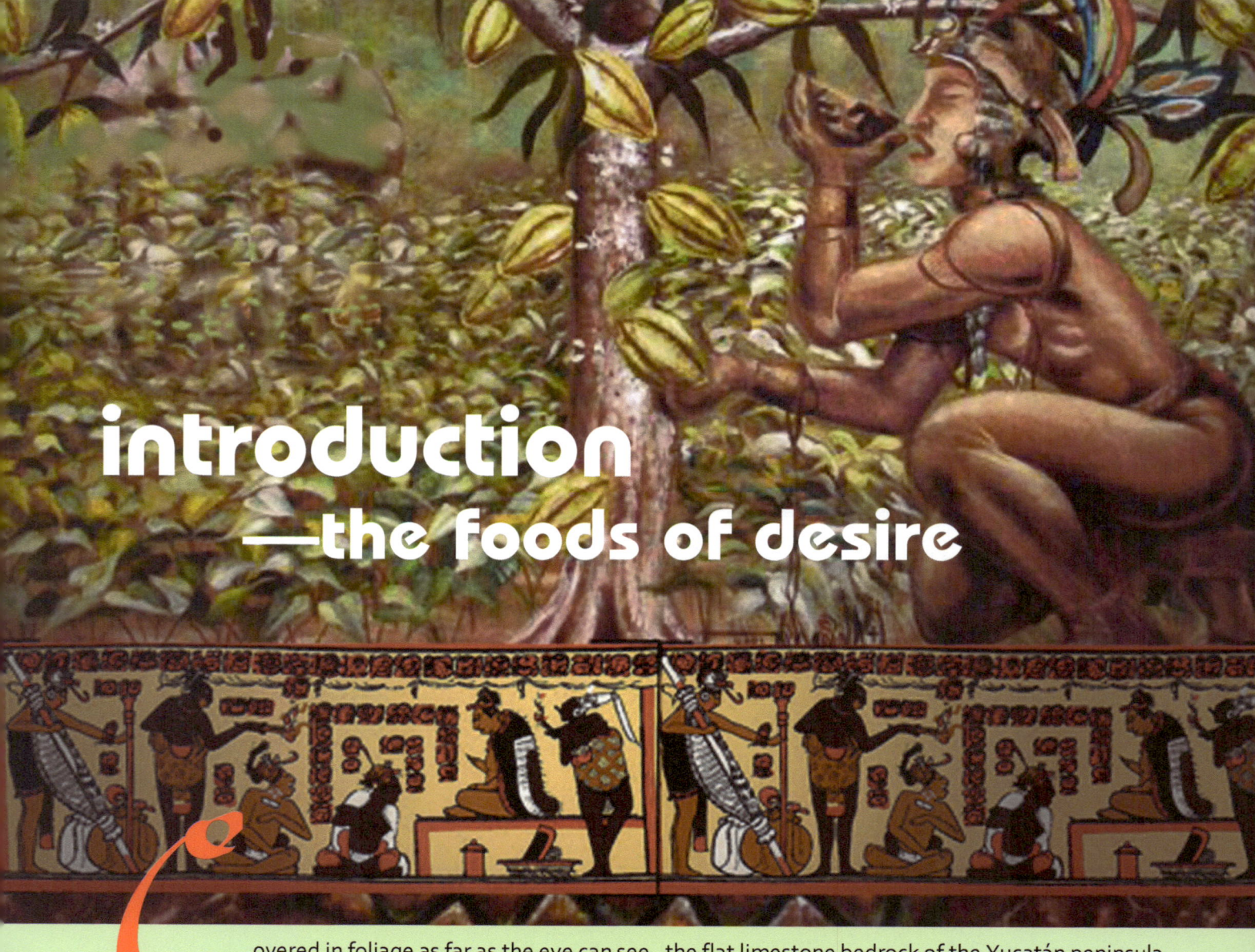

introduction
—the foods of desire

Covered in foliage as far as the eye can see, the flat limestone bedrock of the Yucatán peninsula forms a vast carpet of forest canopy.

Clouds gather. Lightning strikes. Fires burn. Nitrogen from the soil, either as nitrate aerosol or nitrogen oxides gas, is released. The ground becomes more fertile. Seeds yield bountiful harvests.

From the masculine sky a bolt of life strikes the feminine earth and life springs forth. A metaphor is born.

Yes, fertility and food are linked.

Among the Maya, corn harvesting became a ritual, highly symbolic of sex. The phallic-shaped cob was harvested. The husk, resembling foreskin, had to be retracted; seeds of nourishment (life) spilled forth. Throughout the vast ceremonial centers of Maya city-states cults devoted to the power of the phallus were not uncommon. At Uxmal, the Temple of the Phallus celebrates this metaphor. A vast number of phallic sculptures were placed in various positions. Most suggest the earth being fertilized by mankind's toiling of the soil.

Cacao trees are tended. Cacao pods are harvested. Pods are gathered. They are opened. The seeds of these wombs are collected. They are prized above all other things the forests yield.

Chocolate becomes an elixir of desire.

There are rituals associated with the harvests. Cacao beans are protected as a source of wealth. They are prepared as a frothy drink to excite the libido and often consumed during religious ceremonies and festivals.

The elite indulge one another with their ability to secure cacao for themselves and to bestow the luxury of chocolate on their guests.

The feminine power of the earth is embodied in the pleasure of chocolate and in its exhilarating power of virility and fertility.

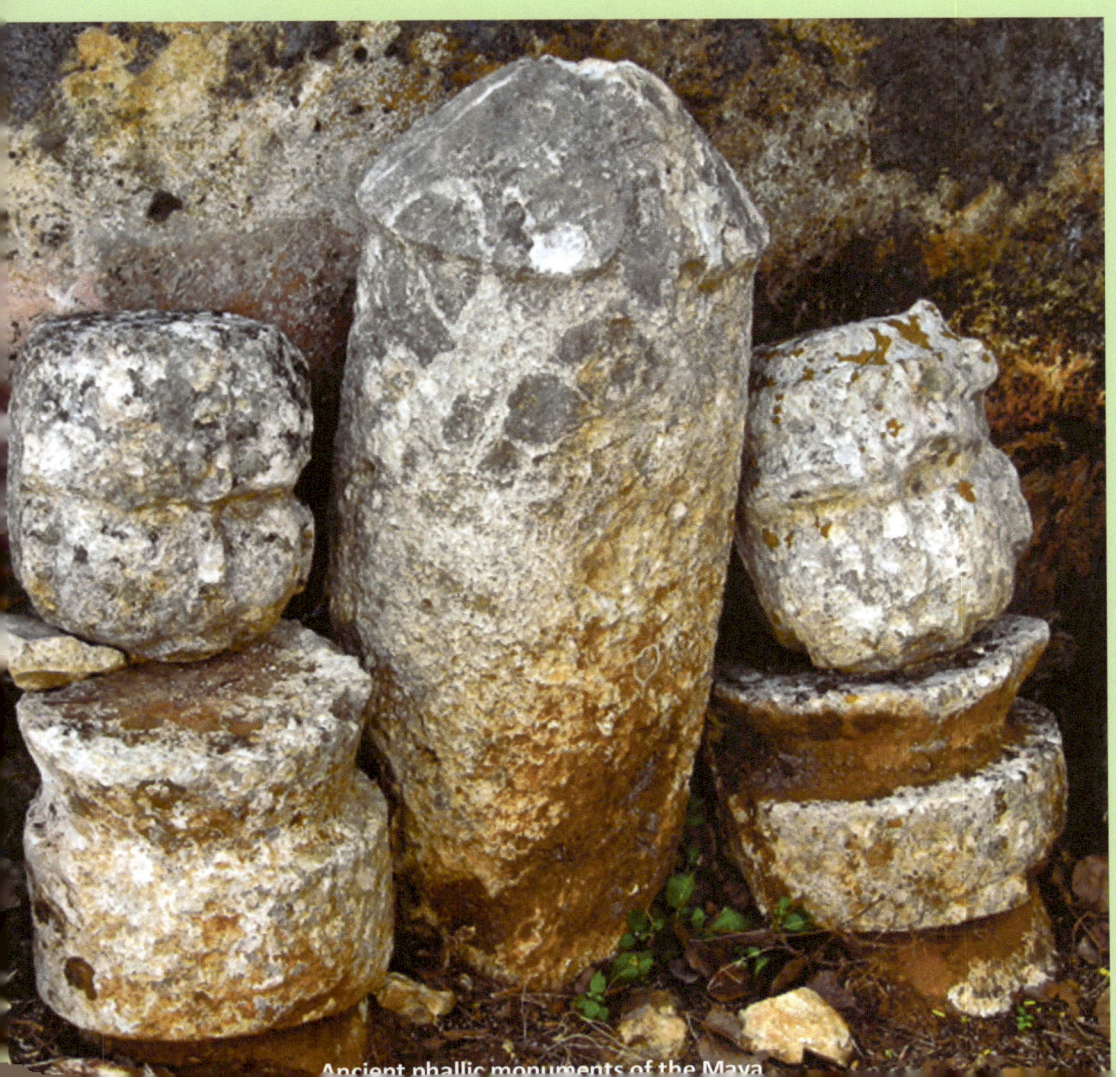

Ancient phallic monuments of the Maya

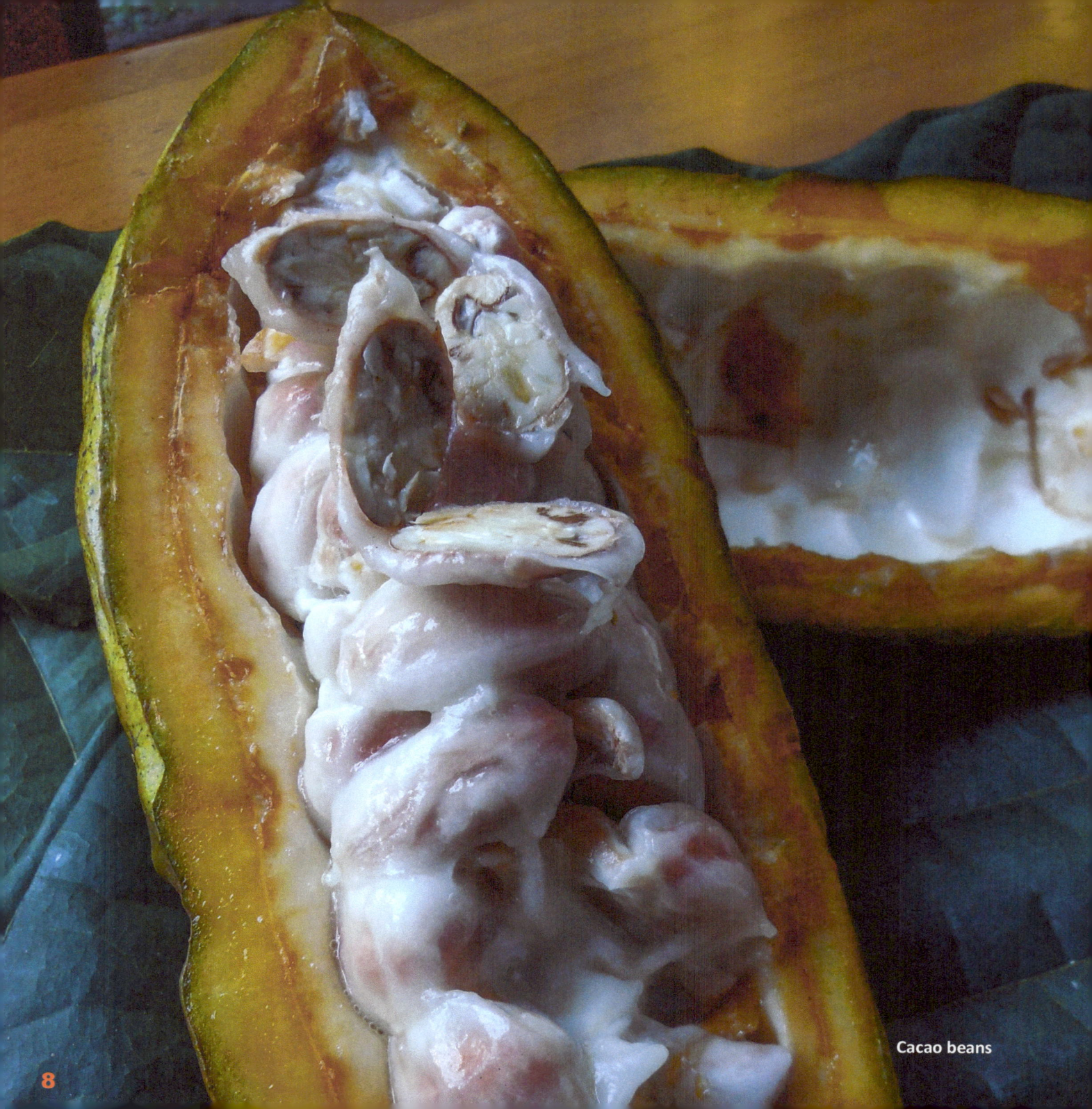
Cacao beans

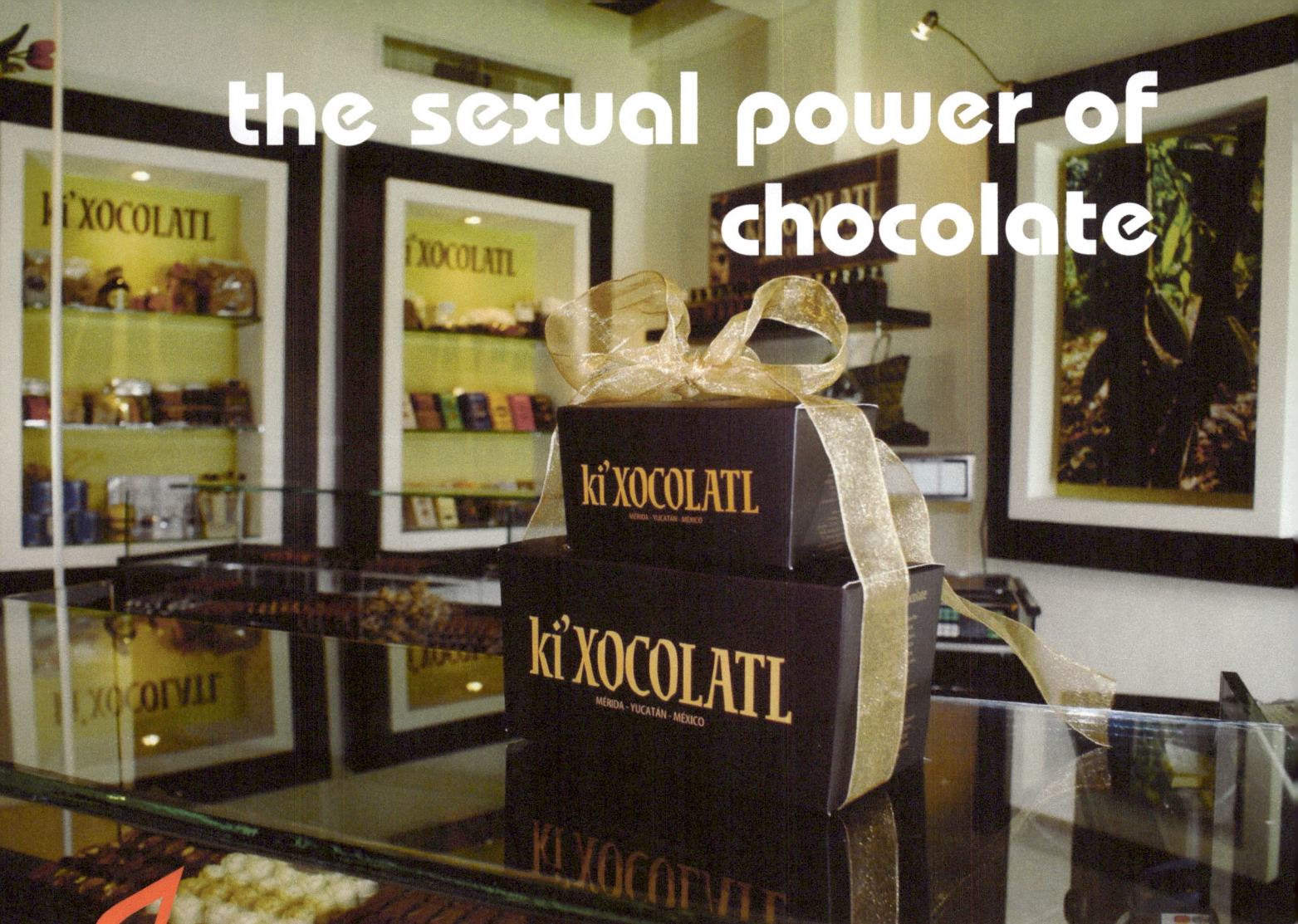

the sexual power of chocolate

It is in the pursuit of desire that chocolate was invented. Yes, I know. You thought chocolate grew on trees. It doesn't. Cacao beans grow on trees, but chocolate? Ah, there it is! Chocolate doesn't grow on trees.

Chocolate was born of human desire. Only once it was imagined by the human mind could it then become a reality in the natural world. Yes, chocolate may be physically derived from cacao beans, but chocolate is the product of countless generations of trial and error, of experimentation, of deliberate thought designed to steal the Secrets of Nature. These are secrets contained in the extraordinary chemical compounds found in the cacao bean. It is through the careful, calculated, and exacting theft of these secrets that humanity was able to invent a food that enhances our sexual desire. Prometheus gave mankind fire. The Mesoamerican people gave the world chocolate. For these gifts both deserve to be venerated.

If chocolate is nourishment worthy for the gods—then it is sustenance for the loves in our lives. Chocolate, you must understand, is more than the food of the gods: it nourishes sex. It is desire. It is lust. It is sex.

Sex.

In the natural evolution of human societies, where there is scarcity, cultural norms evolved in which a man could have as many wives and children as he could materially support. Where there was natural abundance, however, a man could have as many wives as he could . . . sexually satisfy.

Consider the differences in the evolution of human societies over the millennia. In the desert habitats of the Middle East, where an oasis is life, scarcity and the pursuit of resources defined societies. Scarcity also shaped European civilization, which, based on religious beliefs, pursued resources relentlessly around the world.

But what of the tropics? What of lands where life is thrust upon life and people lived in abundance amid verdant gardens of Eden? What of habitats where fragrant flora and bountiful fauna are almost without limit?

What of societies that evolved amid abundance? What of human communities able to indulge in the pursuit of the perfect orgasm?

Sex and chocolate. Chocolate and sex. They are one and the same.

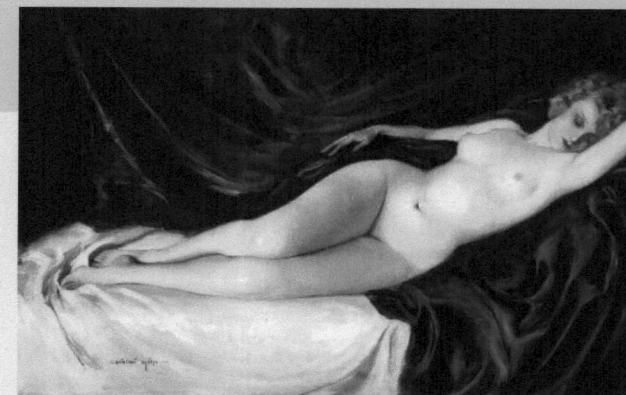

Chocolate, you must understand, was a food invented in mankind's pursuit of the perfect orgasm.

Orgasms and chocolate. Chocolate and orgasms. They are one and the same.

Or they might as well be one and the same.

Perhaps that's why lovers pursue chocolate.

Perhaps that's why the celibate—Catholic nuns and Franciscan friars—substitute chocolate for sexual intercourse.

Perhaps that's why chocolate has been bound by a world of dream, greeted by a lonely heart, a promise.

Across oceans and centuries, even before humanity had a name for the essence in the cacao bean, we, as a species, instinctively sought it out . . . a food, a nutrient, a substance that would defy the physical limits of desire . . .

It became a food that would first nourish and then ignite the loins . . .

It became sustenance that would fuel desire and transcend the natural order of things where ecstasy is concerned . . .

That chocolate can enhance human sexual performance has long been mocked as unfounded superstitions with no basis in fact. In 1996, for instance, Michael Coe completed a manuscript left unfinished when his wife died. It is considered an authoritative book on chocolate.

In *The True History of Chocolate* he writes:

> Psychologists tend to dismiss the possibility that any one of the myriad chemical compounds that constitute chocolate, or any combination of them, could have a physical effect on the consumer. . . . The views of the medical profession on chocolate vary wildly. Some doctors claim it to be an anti-depressant . . . Others can find no such effect. The most extensive medical study of chocolate is by a French doctor, Hervé Robert, who published a book in 1990 called Les virtue thérapeutiques du chocolat. He finds that the caffeine, theobromine, serotonin, and phenylethylamine that chocolate contains make it a tonic, and an anti-depressive and anti-stress agent, enhancing pleasurable activities, including making love.[1]

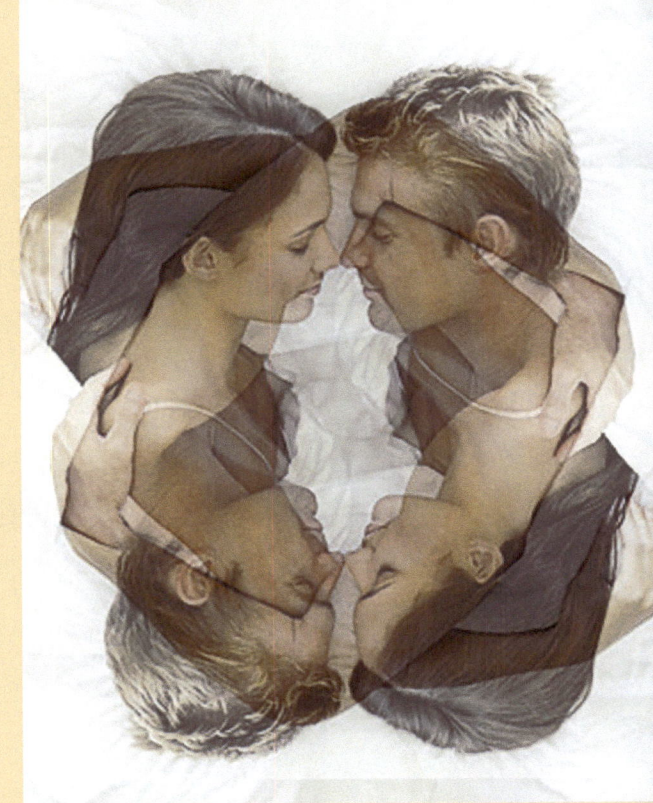

Michael Coe then explains that serotonin, produced naturally in the brain, is a hormone that improves our moods. He continues to elucidate that phynylethylamine is also a naturally-occurring chemical produced in the brain that improves our moods.

Because chocolate contains chemicals associated with feeling good, it might put us in a better frame of mind and make us more willing to engage in love-making.

That's about all he is prepared to concede.

But he is mistaken: chocolate ignites the loins!

In all fairness to Michael Coe, the year that *The True History of Chocolate* was published is the same year that Pfizer patented a medicine designed to produce nitric oxide in the human body. Two years later, the Food and Drug Administration, or FDA, an agency of the U.S. federal government, authorized Pfizer to sell their pharmaceutical to the public.

Its name?

Viagra.

Its purpose?

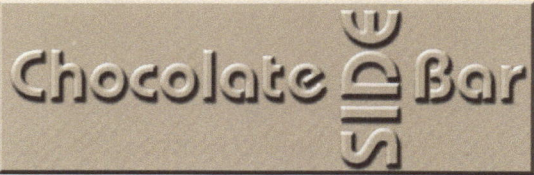

L-Arginine is Essential
Among its Many Roles:

- Is a precursor of nitric oxide (NO)
- Promotes circulation resulting in improved blood flow
- Stimulates the release of growth hormones
- Increases muscle mass, while reducing body fat
- Supports male fertility, improving sperm production and motility
- Reduces risk of blood clots and stroke
- Supports normal blood pressure
- Improves vascular function for patients with angina
- Helps recovery after heart attack
- Helps prevent and treat cardiovascular disease
- Helps reduce growth of cancerous tumors[1]

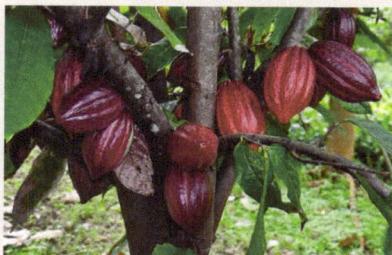

A medication to treat erectile dysfunction.

It's time to dispense with the niceties: chocolate contains arginine, an amino acid found naturally-occurring in the cacao bean. This amino acid is necessary for the production of nitric oxide, which, in turn, stimulates blood flow. In the human male, nitric oxide allows the penile shaft to become engorged with blood, allowing for firmer erections that last longer than they otherwise would. In the human female, nitric oxide allows for the clitoris to become engorged with blood, heightening sensitivity, and enhancing female sexual response.

In both sexes "erections" are heightened, allowing for longer sexual sessions.

Across the ages, the First Peoples of Mesoamerica—the area lying south of the Valley of Mexico and north of Costa Rica—cultivated a tree whose fruit bore a bean possessed by an elixir of substances which, together, excite the mind and empower the physical.

Now consider that holistic practitioners treat erectile dysfunction in men and frigidity in women with arginine supplements, the most readily accessible being chocolate. Both erectile dysfunction and frigidity are considered forms of hypoactive sexual desire disorder (HSDD). Many holistic practitioners argue that pharmaceuticals for treating sexual dysfunction in both men and women can be substituted with L-Arginine supplements. The reason for this claim is that natural sources of arginine also increase the human body's ability to produce nitric oxide.

The more nitric oxide in your body, the better orgasms you are capable of enjoying.

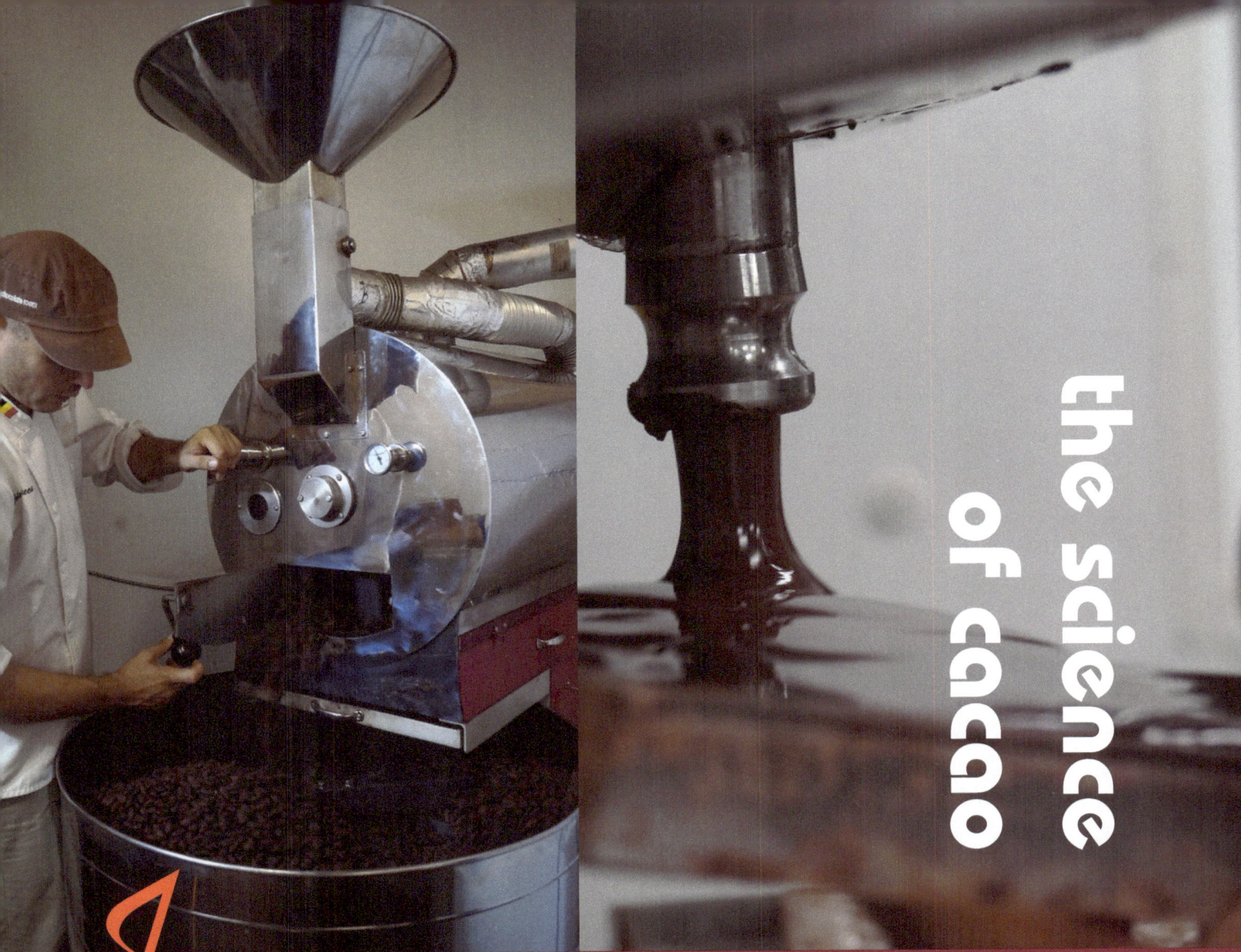

the science of cacao

In the years since the publication of *The True History of Chocolate* scores of scientific studies around the world have established the link between cacao and the production of nitric oxide in the human body. Most of these studies sought to illuminate the role of nitric oxide not on human sexual performance but on cardiovascular disease, congestive heart failure (CHF), and high blood pressure.

Consider a few of the findings:

"Flavanols found in cocoa have been shown to increase the formation of endothelial nitric oxide which promotes vasodilation and therefore blood pressure reduction," from a study, "Effect of Cocoa on Blood Pressure," published in Australia.[2]

"Flavonoid-rich dark chocolate improves endothelial function and is associated with an increase in plasma epicatechin concentrations in healthy adults," concluded a San Francisco, California study titled, "Flavonoid-Rich Dark Chocolate Improves Endothelial Function and Increases Plasma Epicatechin Concentrations in Healthy Adults."[3]

"Dark chocolate and flavonoid-rich cocoa may have a blood pressure-lowering effect. These effects can be attributed to flavonoids and are mainly mediated through increased nitric oxide bioavailability," a study titled "Effect of Dark Chocolate on Arterial Function in Healthy Individuals: Cocoa Instead of Ambrosia?" published in Greece, determined.[4]

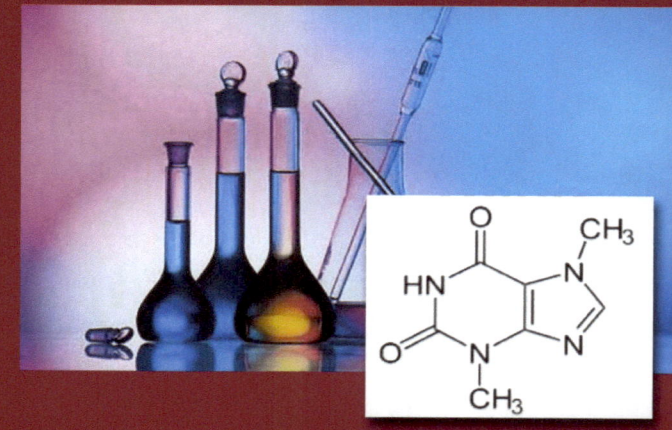

"These data suggest that consumption of chocolate is inversely related with prevalent CHD in a general United States population," a study titled "Chocolate Consumption is Inversely Associated with Prevalent Coronary Heart Disease: The National Heart, Lung, and Blood Institute Family Heart Study," at the Harvard Medical School, concluded.[5]

"Cocoa flavonoids are able to reduce cardiovascular risk by improving endothelial function and decreasing blood pressure (BP)," researchers in a study titled "Blood Pressure and Cardiovascular Risk: What About Cocoa and Chocolate?" published in Italy, confirmed.[6]

"In prehypertension subjects, dark chocolate 30 g/day increased NOx serum levels and decreased systolic blood pressure after 15 days of treatment," concluded an Indonesian study titled "Effect of Dark Chocolate on Nitric Oxide Serum Levels and Blood Pressure in Prehypertension Subjects."[7]

"Containing flavonoids, cacao and its products have antioxidant, anti-inflammatory, anti-atherogenic, anti-thrombotic, antihypertensive and neuroprotective effects, as well as influence on insulin sensitivity, vascular endothelial function, and activation of nitric oxide," a Swiss study titled "Sexuality, Heart and Chocolate," concluded.[8]

"Several potential mechanisms through which cocoa might exert its positive effects have been proposed, among them activation of nitric oxide synthase, increased bioavailability of nitric oxide as well as antioxidant, and anti-inflammatory properties," stated another study from Switzerland titled "Cocoa, Blood Pressure, and Vascular Function."[9]

"This study is the first to identify beneficial vascular effects of flavanol-rich cocoa consumption in hypercholesterolemic postmenopausal women," a study titled "Chronic Consumption of Flavanol-Rich Cocoa

Improves Endothelial Function and Decreases Vascular Cell Adhesion Molecule in Hypercholesterolemic Postmenopausal Women," conducted at the University of California, Davis, concluded.[10]

"This study showed that a short-term intake of dark chocolate might improve the lipoprotein profile in healthy humans, more so in women than in men, and this might exert a protective effect on the cardiovascular system," is the conclusion of a study published in Italy titled "Effect of Consumption of Dark Chocolate on Oxidative Stress in Lipoproteins and Platelets in Women and in Men."[11]

In Spain, a study, titled "The Impact of Chocolate on Cardiovascular Health," determined that "the consumption of chocolate has been involved in the protective modulation of blood pressure, the lipid profile, the activation of platelets, and the sensitivity to insulin."[12]

"The mechanisms underlying these responses are likely diverse, however most data suggest an effect of increased nitric oxide bioavailability," a study titled "Effect of Cocoa/Chocolate Ingestion on Brachial Artery Flow-Mediated Dilation and Its Relevance to Cardiovascular Health and Disease in Humans," published in Hershey, Pennsylvania, concluded. "Thus, positive vascular effects of cocoa/chocolate on the endothelium may underlie (i.e., be linked mechanistically to) reductions in cardiovascular risk in humans."[13]

These are just 12 studies. There are today hundreds of such studies. None contradict the fact that cacao increases nitric oxide production in the human organism. None contradict the expectation that this is instrumental for superior sexual performance. What is important for the discussion presented here is that modern science is fast confirming the importance of cacao in producing nitric oxide in the human body.

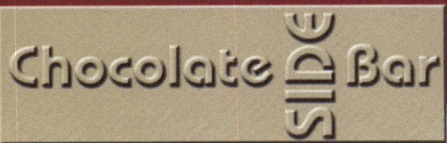

A Nobel Prize for Your Efforts

One would think that this discovery is of such importance that it is worthy of a Nobel Prize.

Guess what?

It is!

In case you missed it, in 1998 the Nobel Prize in Physiology (Medicine) was awarded to Robert F. Furchgott, Louis J. Ignarro, and Ferid Murad for their discoveries that nitric oxide, or NO, is a signaling molecule. The official announcement declared: "We know today that NO acts as a signal molecule in the nervous system and as a gate keeper of blood flow to different organs. . . . This can modulate many functions."

Yes.

Many functions: Stronger erections. Flushed clitorises. More vigorous orgasms. The Maya knew this. And upon the Nobel committee confirming it to be so, a prize was awarded. A Nobel Prize for the Sexual Power of Chocolate.

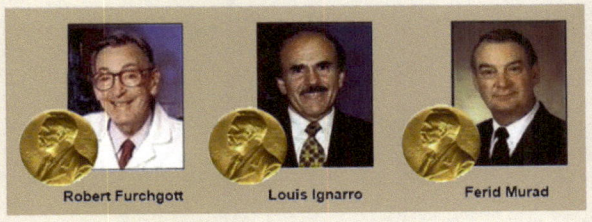

the varietals of cacao beans

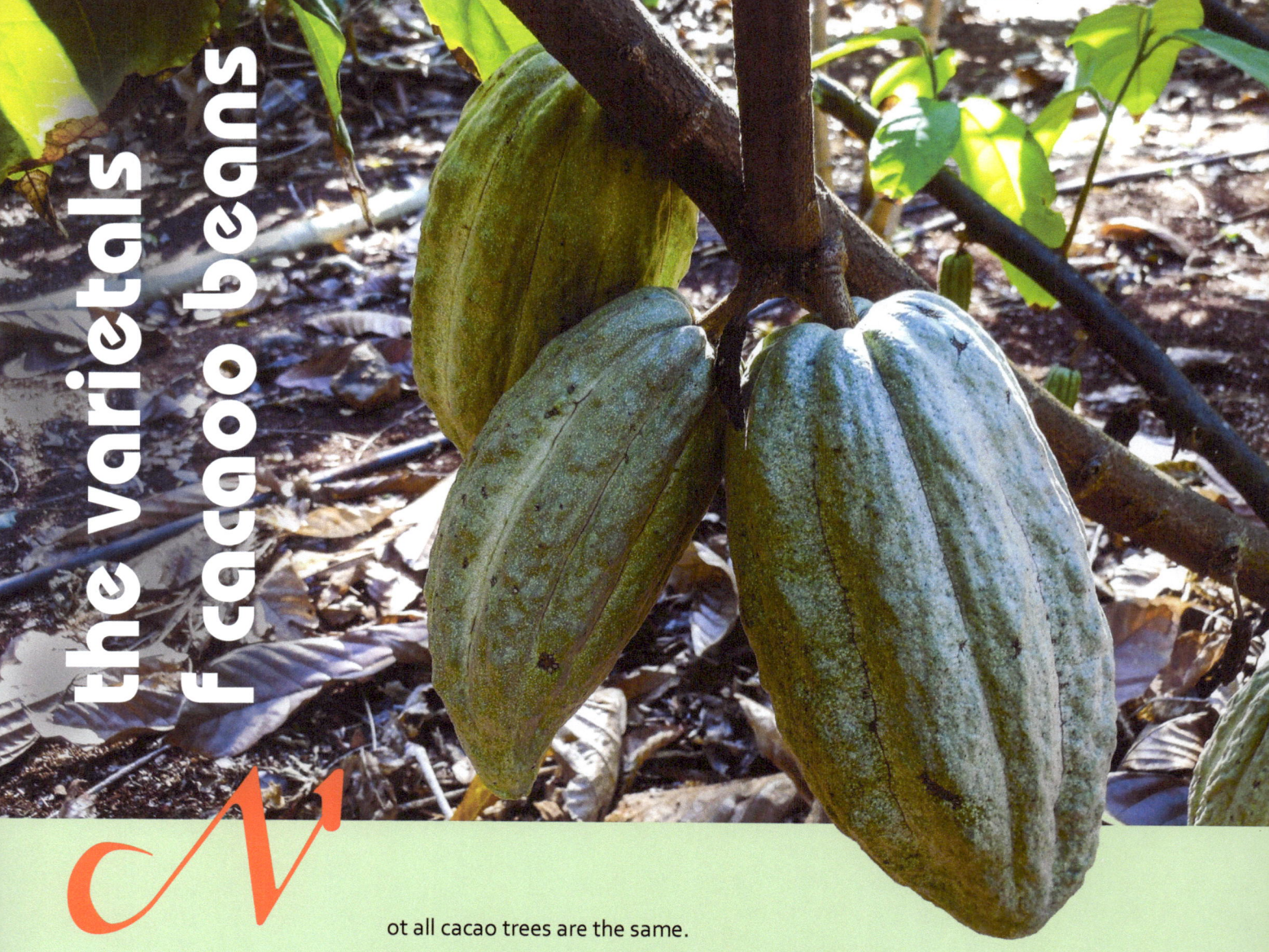

Not all cacao trees are the same.

If I were to tell you that there's a difference between grape juice and a bottle of fine wine, I'm confident that you would agree with me without a moment's hesitation. There is, after all, quite a difference between having a glass of Welch's grape juice and a glass of 2009 Dominus Estate Cabernet Sauvignon!

Yes, both are derived from *grapes*, but what a difference!

The same holds true for chocolates.

There are three cacao varieties and there's a world of difference in the kinds of chocolates that are derived from them—at least when it comes to human sexuality.

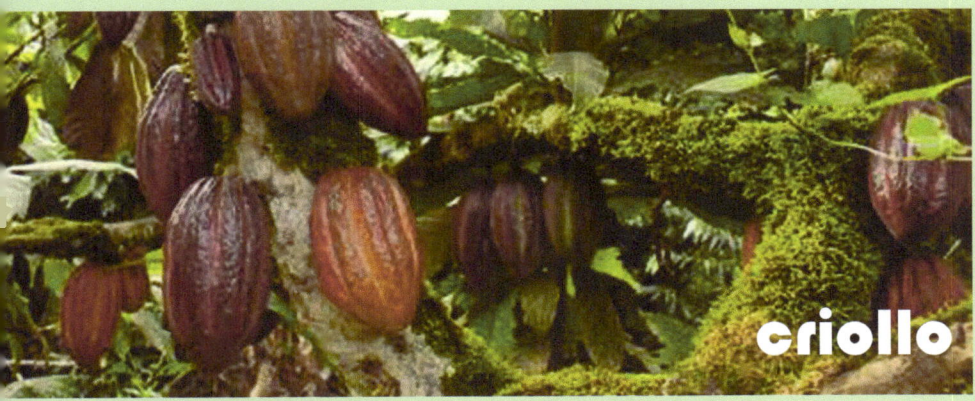

The premium cacao bean, representing less than 2 percent of the world's production, is *criollo*. Superior chocolates are made from the criollo cacao bean. Its scarcity is a result of the delicate nature of the criollo cacao tree. It requires constant care, nurturing, and it yields far fewer cacao fruit than other varieties. The criollo cacao tree requires a constant gardener to lavish thoughtful care on it. It is the criollo cacao that the ancient peoples of Mesoamerica pursued with an abiding passion. Its aroma, flavor, and ability to enhance human sexual response elevated this variety to its exalted position in their cultures. Criollo cacao is believed to contain the more complex cornucopia of chemicals, which together, affect a person's mood, heightens the senses, and unleashes a series of physical changes that enhances human sexual performance.

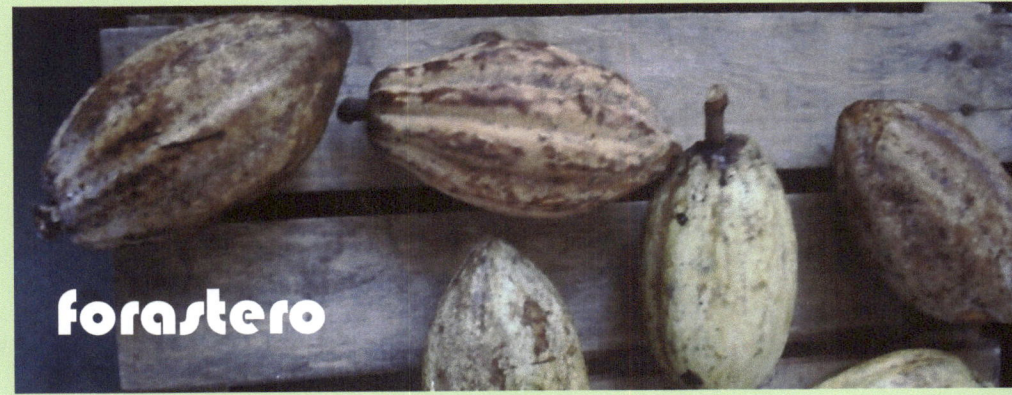

This hardier and more abundant variety represents more than 85 percent of world's cacao production. Grown almost exclusively in West Africa, chocolatiers find this the more commercial cacao variety. On international markets, forastero beans are bought by the ton, and shipped the world over to ports in Europe, the Americas, and Asia. It is the cacao used to produce mass market chocolate for multitudes of consumers. Now for the bad news: forastero cacao from West Africa is part of the "conflict cacao" market. Given contemporary sensibilities and interest in social justice, many consumers are concerned about the conditions under which the foods they consume are produced. Much of West African cacao is produced through a system that condemns workers to lives of poverty and exploitation. In *Bitter Chocolate,* author Carol Off documents the worker exploitation that characterizes the forastero plantations of West Africa. "Carol Off draws an even more sordid picture of the relationship between the institution of slavery and the rise of British chocolate capitalism under such magnates as Cadbury," Mark Knoblauch writes in Booklist. "Worse still, Carol Off asserts, slavery continues to be a vexing, intractable problem in these West African regions."

The book in your hands does not recommend any "conflict cacao" without identifying it as such.

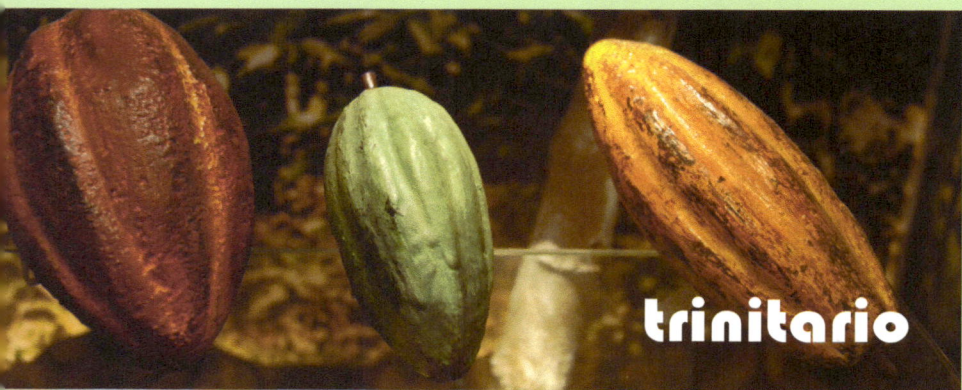

For centuries, hybridizers have sought to create a cacao variety that combines the flavor, aroma, and delicacy of the criollo cacao bean with the sturdiness and yield of the foraster cacao bean. Beginning in the eighteenth century, on the island of Trinidad in the Caribbean, commercial interests endeavored to use cross-pollination to invent such a variety. The result is the trinitario cacao bean. Today, it constitutes approximately 15 percent of the world's production, more often found throughout the Caribbean and Central America. This variety, somewhat more expensive than forastero, faces commercial resistance on the world markets, which is designed to reward the least expensive cacao bean. Trinitario, however, has a superior flavor and aroma than forastero. It cannot, however, compete with the excellence of the criollo bean.

Having now addressed the differences among the varietals of cacao beans, we can proceed to discuss the ideal chocolate capable of delivering superior sexual performance. First, I will dispense with forastero cacao. Why? Because, you, gentle reader, deserve superior cacao.

You are worthy of extraordinary sex. You will delight in spectacular orgasms. For these same reasons I will also dispense with trinitario cacao. A hybrid cacao varietal, for you and your sex life, simply won't do. A hybrid cacao will not deliver the spectacular orgasm you deserve. Leave this for the limp-dick drug addicts and frigid-anorgasmic women the world over. You are above such a fate. With forastero and trinitario both disqualified . . .

That leaves criollo cacao.

Criollo Reigns Supreme. It is settled. The matter is now concluded. For you, gentle reader, only the best will do.

Criollo. Criollo cacao. Chocolate made from criollo cacao.

Only criollo cacao bursts with all the chemicals—arginine, caffeine, theobromine, serotonin, and phenylethylamine—that constitute the elixir for increased sexual performance. To settle on a selection of suitable criollo chocolates for increased sexual performance, I, like a modern-day Indiana Jones, had to navigate my way through this virtual Garden of Eden of Chocolates.

I analyzed, scrutinized, sampled, and quantified 282 brands in the course of conducting research and experimentation over a three-year period. You're welcome.

What follows is a description the superior chocolates for extraordinary sex.

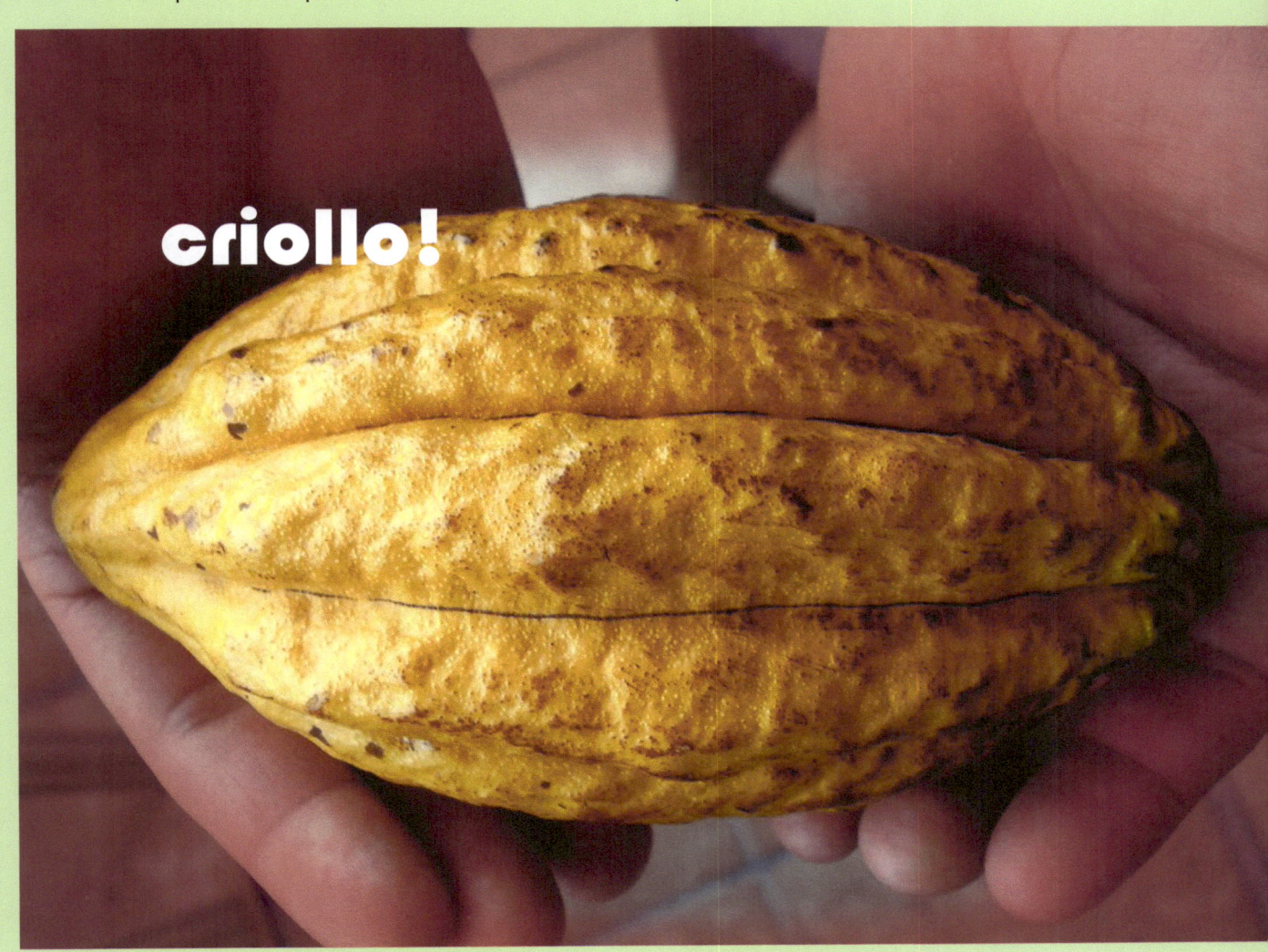

a chocolate regimen for enhanced sexual performance

"The idea of waiting for something makes it more exciting," - Andy Warhol

Here is a recommended dietary regimen for attaining peak human sexual performance through cacao.

Consume 30 to 40 grams (1 to 2 ounces) of chocolate every day. Dark chocolate, 70 percent cacao, or higher, content. It has to be 100 percent criollo cacao.

Individuals who consume dark, criollo chocolate, in the recommended quantities, on average, can begin to enjoy enhanced sexual performance three to six weeks into the regimen.

Stronger Libido . . . Greater Endurance

Higher blood flow makes clitoral and vaginal tissues more sensitive and responsive to sexual stimulation and helps increase the possibility of reaching orgasm. Although there haven't been nearly as many studies done on arginine supplementation in women as in men, one study found that postmenopausal women who took a supplement including L-Arginine experienced heightened sexual response.

Another study involving 77 women of all ages found that after four weeks, 73.percent of the women who took a supplement including L-Arginine experienced greater sexual satisfaction, including heightened desire and clitoral sensation, frequency of intercourse and orgasm, and less vaginal dryness.

—*Sexual dysfunction in the United States: prevalence and predictors*, by Laumann EO, Paik A, and Rosen RC, Department of Sociology, University of Chicago, Illinois.

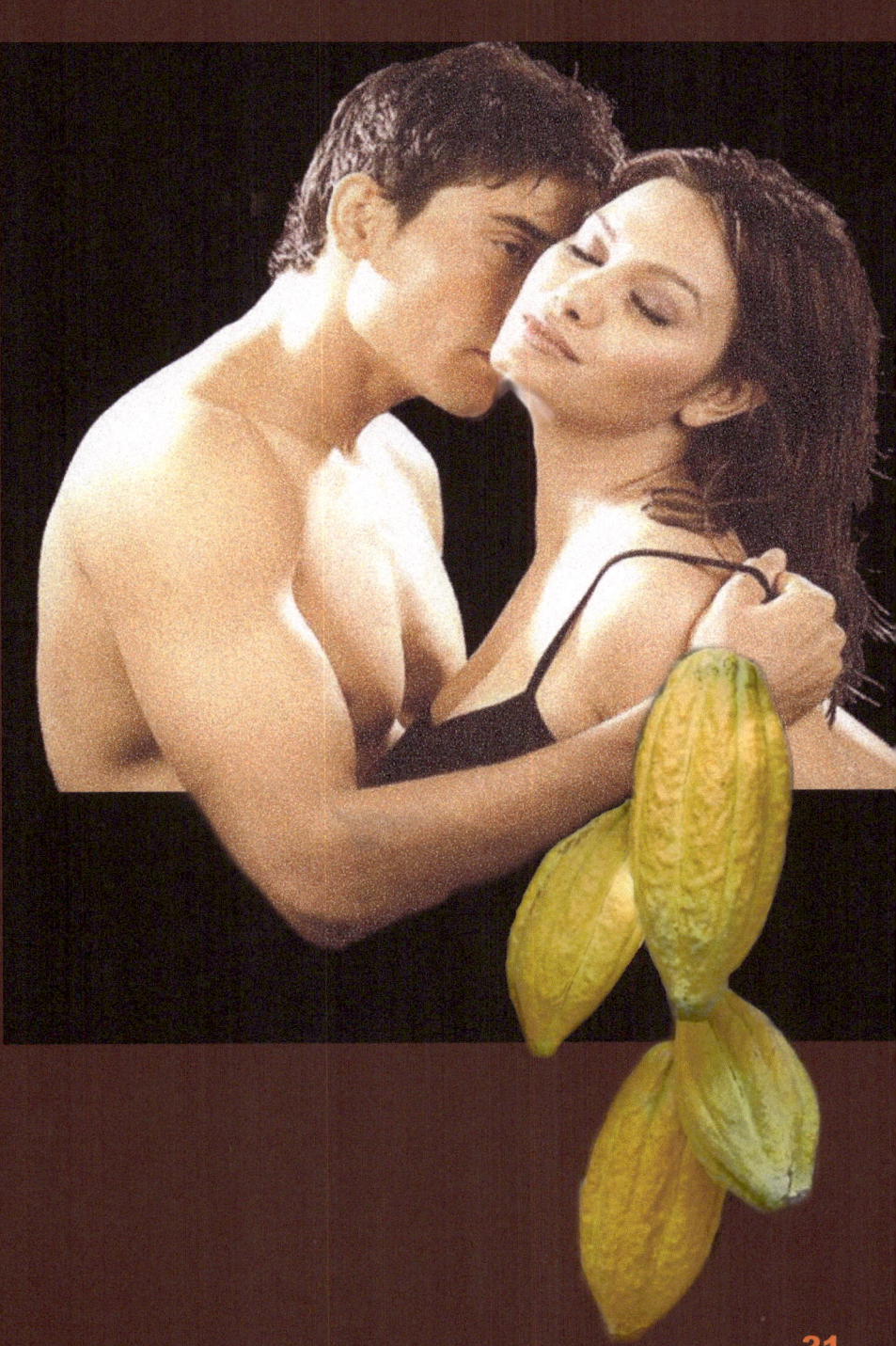

"Slave-Tested, Master-Approved"

What is that thing? I can't remember. Some exclamation or was it a repudiation? Oh, yes, it proclaimed something or other . . . Yes, that's it, a proclamation . . . the Emancipation Proclamation . . . freeing slaves in the Confederate States of America. . .

Then there's that other cumbersome statement from the United Nations General Assembly. You know the one: Article 4 of the Universal Declaration of Human Rights. It reads: "No one shall be held in slavery or servitude; slavery and the slave trade shall be prohibited in all their forms." Tell that to the 200,000+ children forced to work cacao plantations in West Africa!

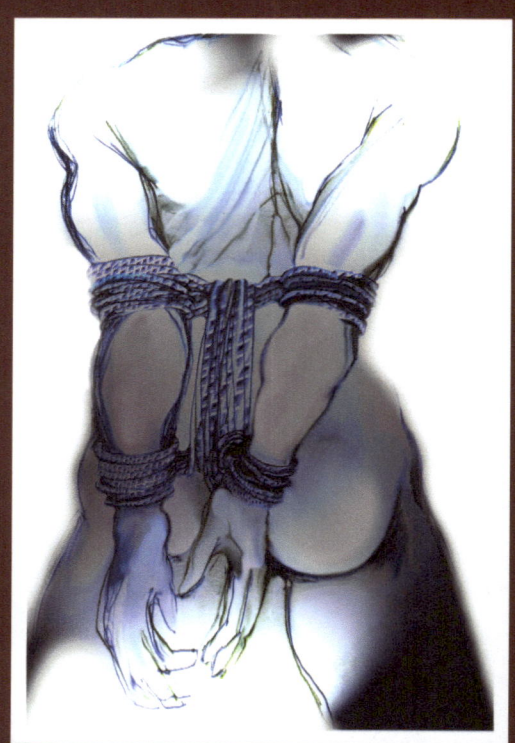

Binding My Muse by Carolyn Weltman

"Some of them want to abuse you / Some of them want to be abused."—Eurythmics

With this caveat, I am confident that you, as I, have been surprised at the proliferation in the number of chapters of the Masters and slaves Together (MAsT) organization throughout the world.

In the realm of voluntary "slavery," which is the world of fetish servitude, sadomasochism, and fantasy sex, there are greater opportunities for scientific inquiry. In the late 1990s I enlisted the assistance of two individuals, who are professionals, in an experiment to test the impact of consuming 100 percent criollo dark chocolate over a period of six weeks on human sexual performance. One was a Mistress who operates a dungeon on 10th Street between Fifth Avenue and Avenue of the Americas in New York. The other was a Master whose dungeon was on Roosevelt Way, near Clifford Terrace, in San Francisco. Both worked with male and female submissive clients who were into being controlled and dominated.

Both Mistress and Master reported that there were measurable increases in the sexual stamina and performance of the individuals ordered to consume fifty grams (1.7637 ounces) of chocolate every day for a six-week period. The cacao content of the chocolate supplied was 70 percent. It was organic and 100 percent criollo. The 48 men and women who participated in this experiment, furthermore, refrained from drinking more than one glass of wine per day. A glass of wine consists of 150 milliliters (5 ounces). No hard liquor was allowed. Each participant slept between six and eight hours each night.

No other dietary or sleep restrictions were commanded. The Mistress reported that, by her measurements, sexual performance increased an average of 38 percent; the Master reported an increase of 43 percent. Peer review inquiries are welcome.

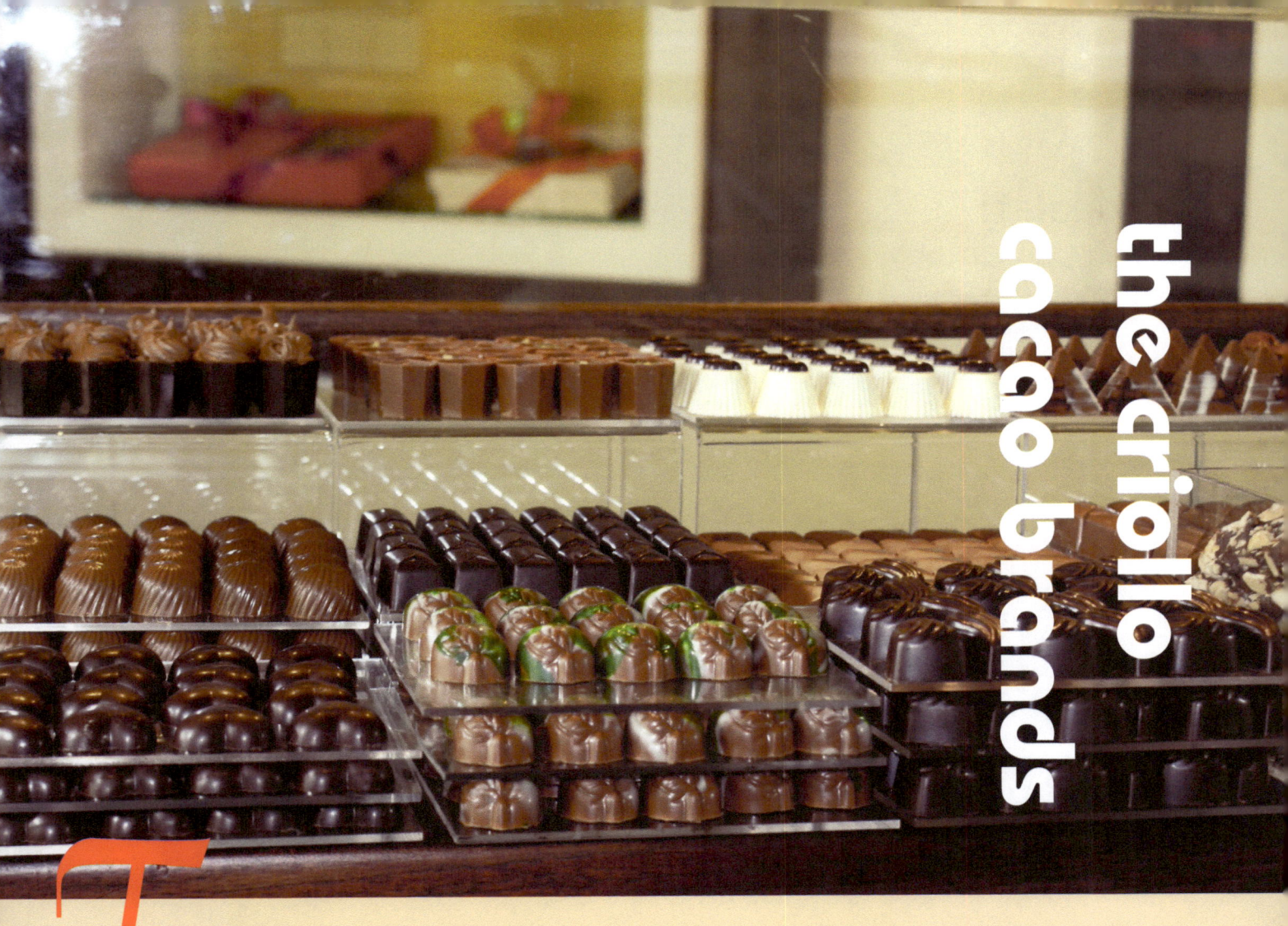

the criollo cacao brands

Forget Madison Avenue marketing. Whether it is Godiva or Jacques Torres, Tolberone or Lindt, Theo Chocolate or Ghirardelli, these are inferior products made from non-criollo cacao beans or from cacao arbitrarily bought from the world market ("conflict cacao").

Chocolate made from cacao of undocumented pedigree will simply never do. Not for you.

Rest assured, however, that the challenge has been met.

What follows are the 100 percent criollo cacao organic chocolates that, in the opinion of this authority, deliver superior sexual performance.[14]

Following are the best 100 percent criollo cacao chocolate bars in the world:

Ki' Xocolatl (Mexico)

100 percent criollo (Mexico)

72 percent cacao

Where to purchase: www.ki-xocolatl.com and www.mexican-chocolate.com

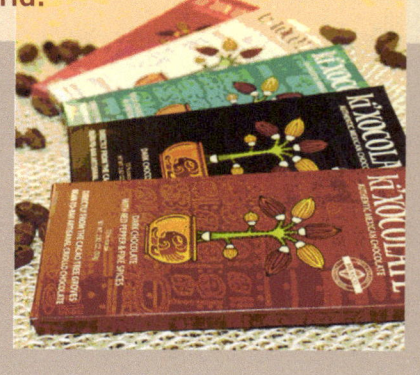

Cacao Prieto (USA)

100 percent criollo (Dominican Republic)

72 percent cacao

Where to purchase: www.cacaoprieto.com

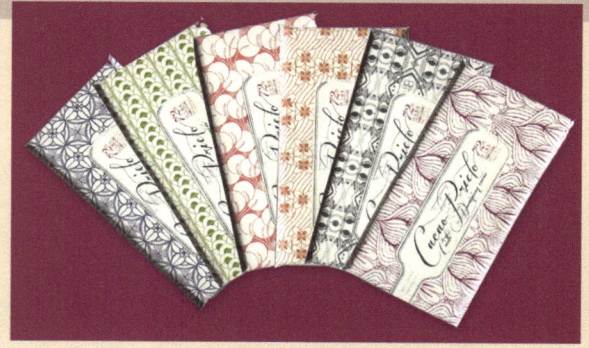

Francois Pralus (Madagascar Criollo) (France)

100 percent criollo (Madagascar)

75 percent cacao

Where to purchase: www.chocolats-pralus.com

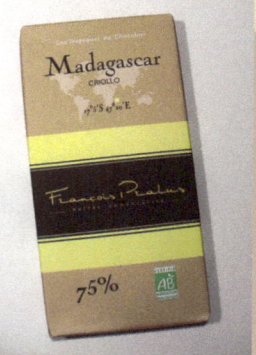

Åkesson's (Switzerland)

100 percent criollo (Madagascar)

75 percent cacao

Where to purchase: www.akessons-organic.com

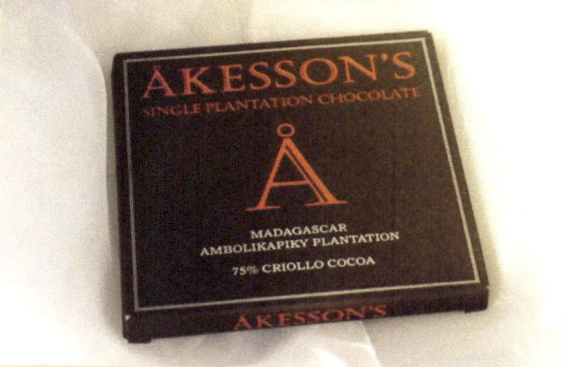

Francois Pralus (France)

100 percent criollo (Indonesia)

75 percent cacao

Where to purchase: *www.chocolats-pralus.com*

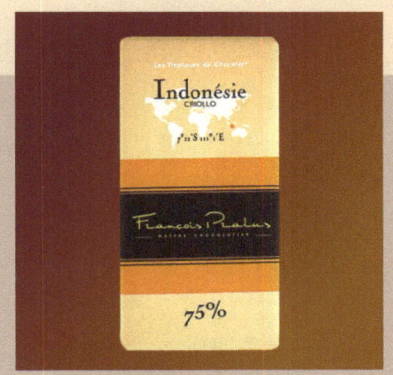

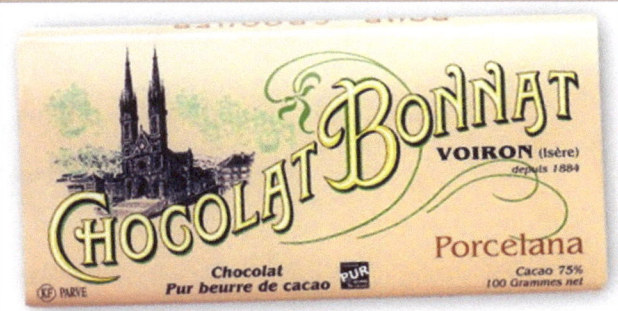

Chocolat Bonnat (Porcelana) (France)

100 percent criollo (Venezuela)

75 percent cacao

Where to purchase: *www.bonnat-chocolatier.com*

Domori Chuao (Italy)

100 percent criollo (Venezuela)

70 percent cacao

Where to purchase: *www.domori.com*

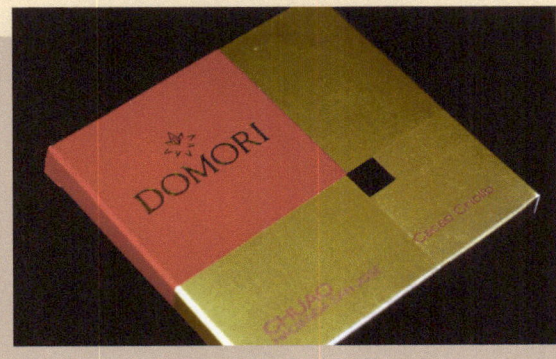

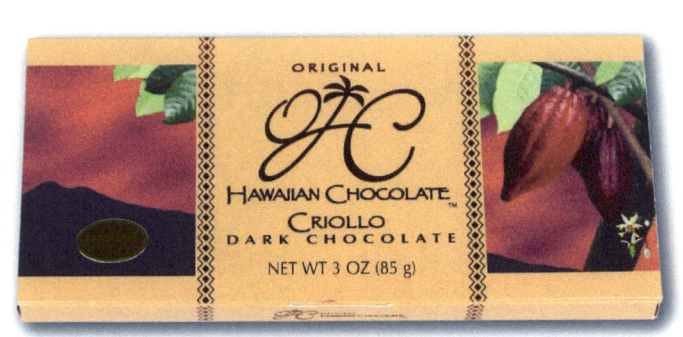

Hawaiian Chocolate (USA)

100 percent criollo (Hawai'i)

70 percent cacao

Where to purchase: *www.ohcf.us*

Royce' 100 percent Criollo (Japan)

100 percent criollo (Venezuela)

Where to purchase: www.e-royce.com

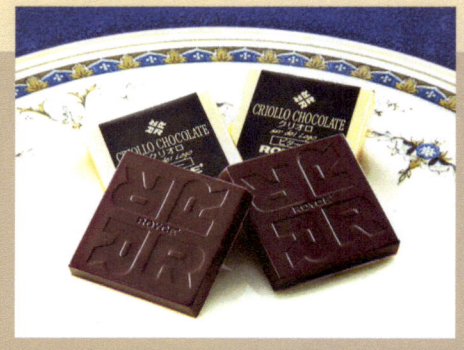

Domori Chuao (Italy)

100 percent criollo (Venezuela)

100 percent cacao

Where to purchase: www.domori.com

Amedei Porcelana (Italy)

100 percent criollo (Venezuela)

70 percent cacao

Where to purchase: www.amedei.com

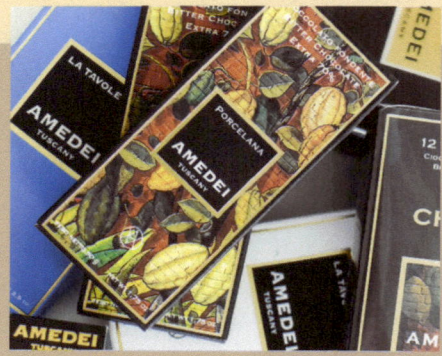

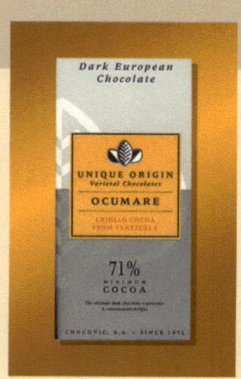

Chocovic (Ocumare) (Spain)

100 percent criollo (Venezuela)

71 percent cacao

Where to purchase: www.chocovic.es

In the preceding list of the recommended 100 percent criollo cacao chocolates from which to choose, please take note of the following:

Only 100 percent criollo cacao chocolates that are organic were listed.

The top five chocolates are made from single-origin producers.

Of the seven that follow the top five, six are produced from criollo cacao originating in Venezuela (one other is Hawaiian). Questions have arisen for the better part of a decade concerning the sociopolitical conditions in Venezuela which may now constitute "conflict cacao." For this reason both Bonnat and Domori were excluded from the top five.

The Dignity of Humanity is more important than any chocolate.

You can enjoy these chocolates knowing that you will derive the full benefits of 100 percent ciollo cacao chocolate without contributing to the exploitation of the most vulnerable members of humanity.

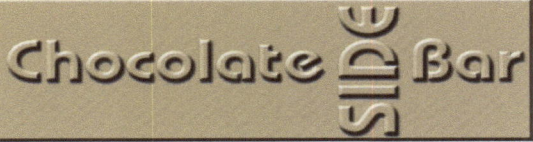

The Lord Cacao

And the Lord Cacao sings, 'I belong in the service of humanity
I belong in the service of procreation
I belong in the service of those whose passion is inflamed
I belong in the service of naked bodies entwined
I belong in the service of humanity
I belong in the tingling of the loins
I belong in the lust of youth
I belong in the climax of naked bodies
I belong more to you than to me!'
   — Song of the Mayab

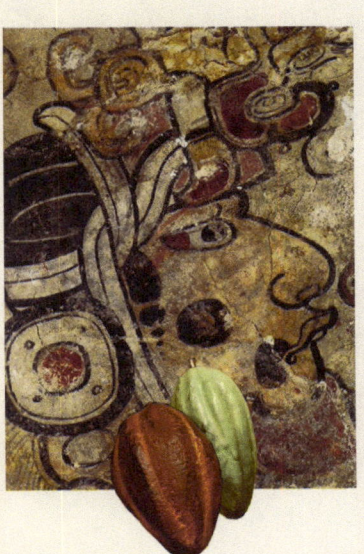

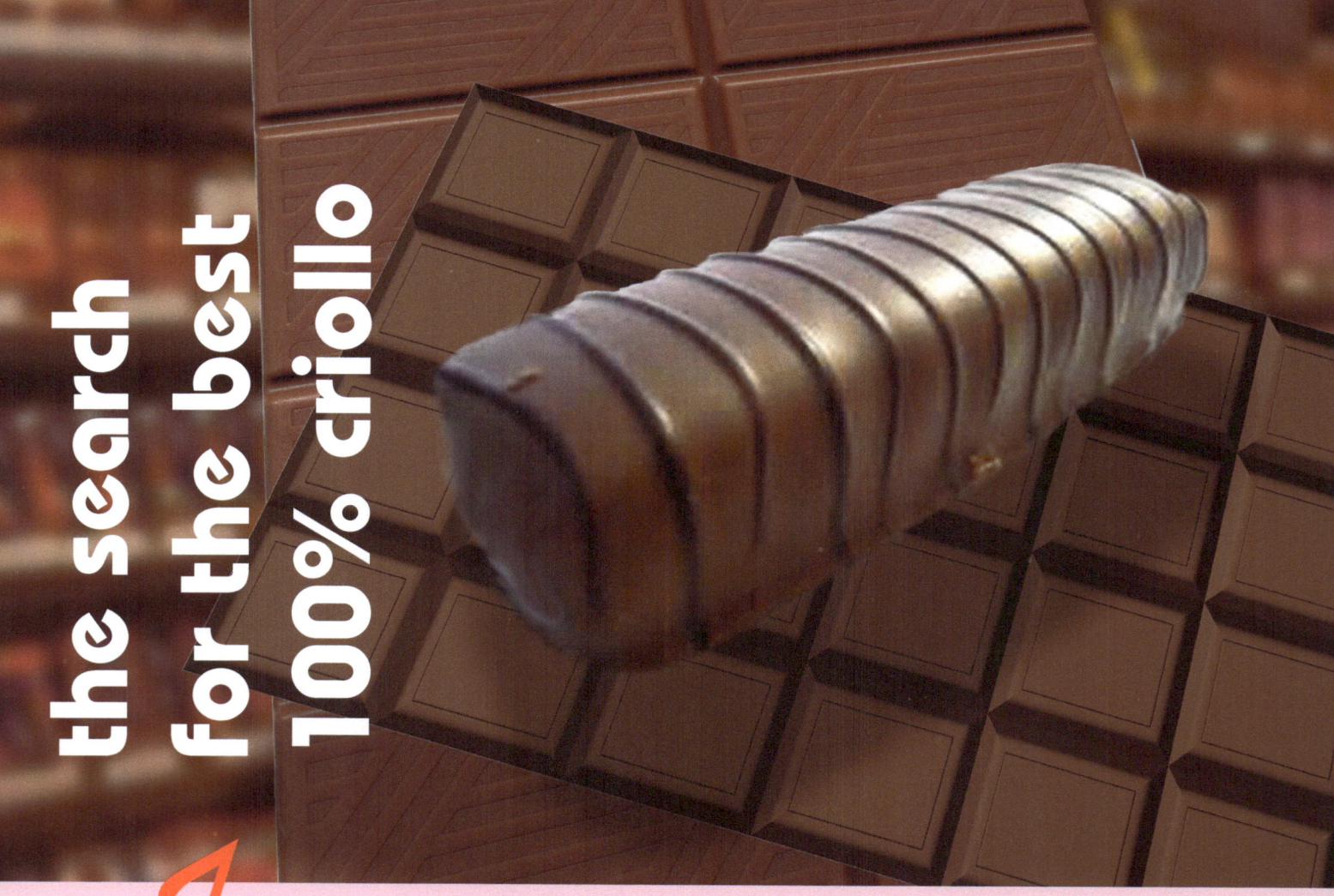

the search for the best 100% criollo

It is not the most prudent thing in the world to argue with Mother Nature.

It is not advisable to challenge master chocolatiers who have earned the right to be included in the *Michelin Guide*.

It is not judicious to pass up an opportunity to wear a pith helmet.

So begins a journey in search of the best 100 percent criollo chocolate in the world.

But truth has to be told: I have an advantage. I've read Dominque Persoone's book, *Cacao: The Roots of Chocolate*. Published in 2009, it was awarded the prestigious Gourmand World Cookbook Award, which declared it "Best Book in the World for Chocolate."

Dominique Persoone embarked on a journey to Mexico in search of chocolate. He ended up in the Yucatán, where he met Mathieu Brees, a fellow Master Chocolatier from Belgium. Mathieu Brees, in turn, had set out to rediscover how the Maya cultivated their criollo cacao and how they made the world's most authentic chocolate. Chocolate, itself the product of generations of constant gardeners who crafted the cacao tree in order to invent a plant capable of producing a food that enhances human sexual response, demands much historical research.

The techniques the early Mesoamericans developed when they took a wild grass and invented corn (maize), after all, are the same skills the Maya subsequently applied to cultivate the cacao tree in order to produce a fruit suitable for the making of chocolate. It is this process, lost across the ages when the Classic Maya civilization collapsed in the tenth century C.E., that had to be reclaimed.

It is Mathieu Brees who, nonetheless, armed with the world-class understanding of chocolate, sought to enlist the Maya people of today as collaborators in a journey to rediscover the Secrets of Nature and their long-distant past.

It is in the heart of the Yucatán, with the same soil, rainfalls, tropical warmth, and environment that first gave the world chocolate as it was prized centuries ago, that had to be reclaimed.

Good news!

After years of dedicated labor, Mathieu Brees has now created an extraordinary line of chocolates that replicate the aphrodisiac properties of 100 percent criollo cacao as the Maya once envisioned and had created: Ki' Xocolatl.

Once lost, it is now rediscovered.

It is born again, in a new and eternal life . . . *of heightened sexual pleasure.*

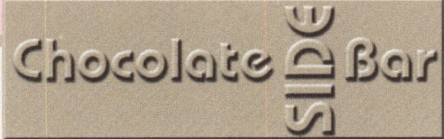

Chocolate Side Bar

Stronger Libido …
Greater Endurance

"Both men and women report that L-Arginine seems to increase their libido or desire for sex, and some also report that L-Arginine gives them greater endurance and stronger, more powerful orgasms. Reports also suggest that L-Arginine supplements can improve fertility in men who have low sperm counts or poor sperm motility (activity)."

See: "Sexual Dysfunction in the United States: Prevalence and Predictors," by Laumann EO, Paik A, and Rosen RC, Department of Sociology, University of Chicago, Illinois.

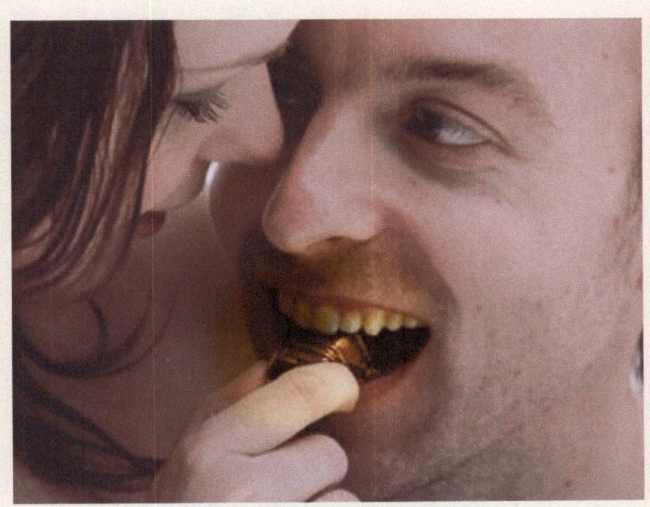

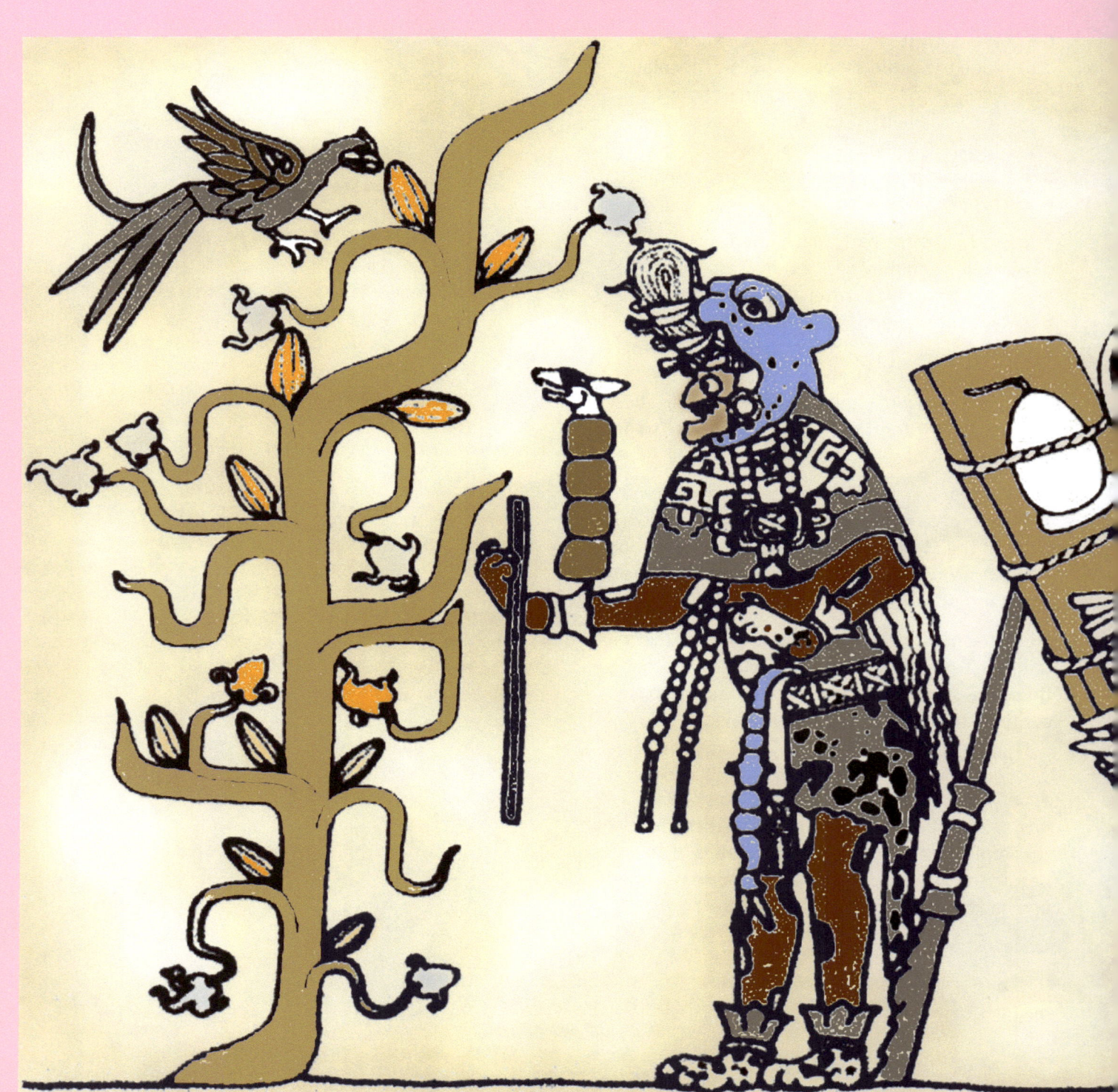

30

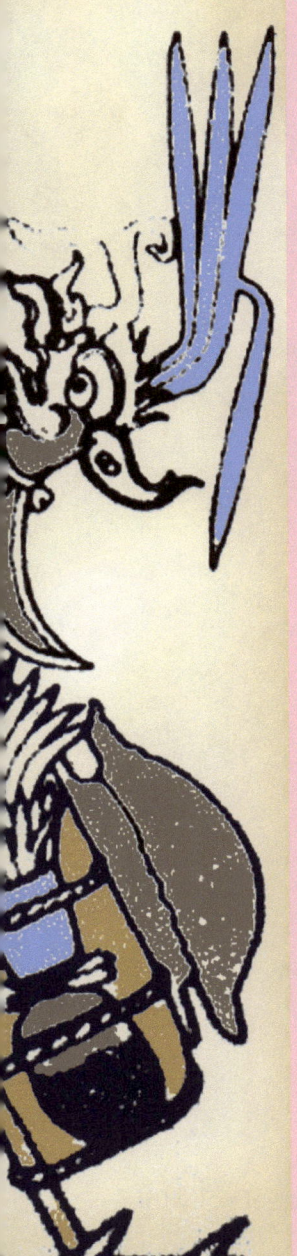

Chocolate Side Bar

It's Good to be Emperor

Aztec Emperor Motecuhzoma Xocoyotzin, also known as Moctezuma II, is believed to have had more than 200 concubines at his command.

From time to time they brought to him some cups of fine gold, with a certain drink made of cacao, which they said was for success with women; and then we thought no more of it; but I saw that they brought more than 50 great jars of prepared good cacao with its foam, and he drank of that; and that the women who served him drink very respectfully . . .
—Bernal Díaz del Castillo, *The True History of the Conquest of New Spain*

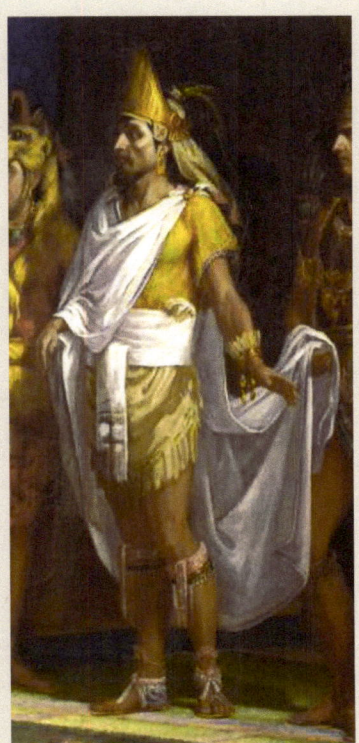

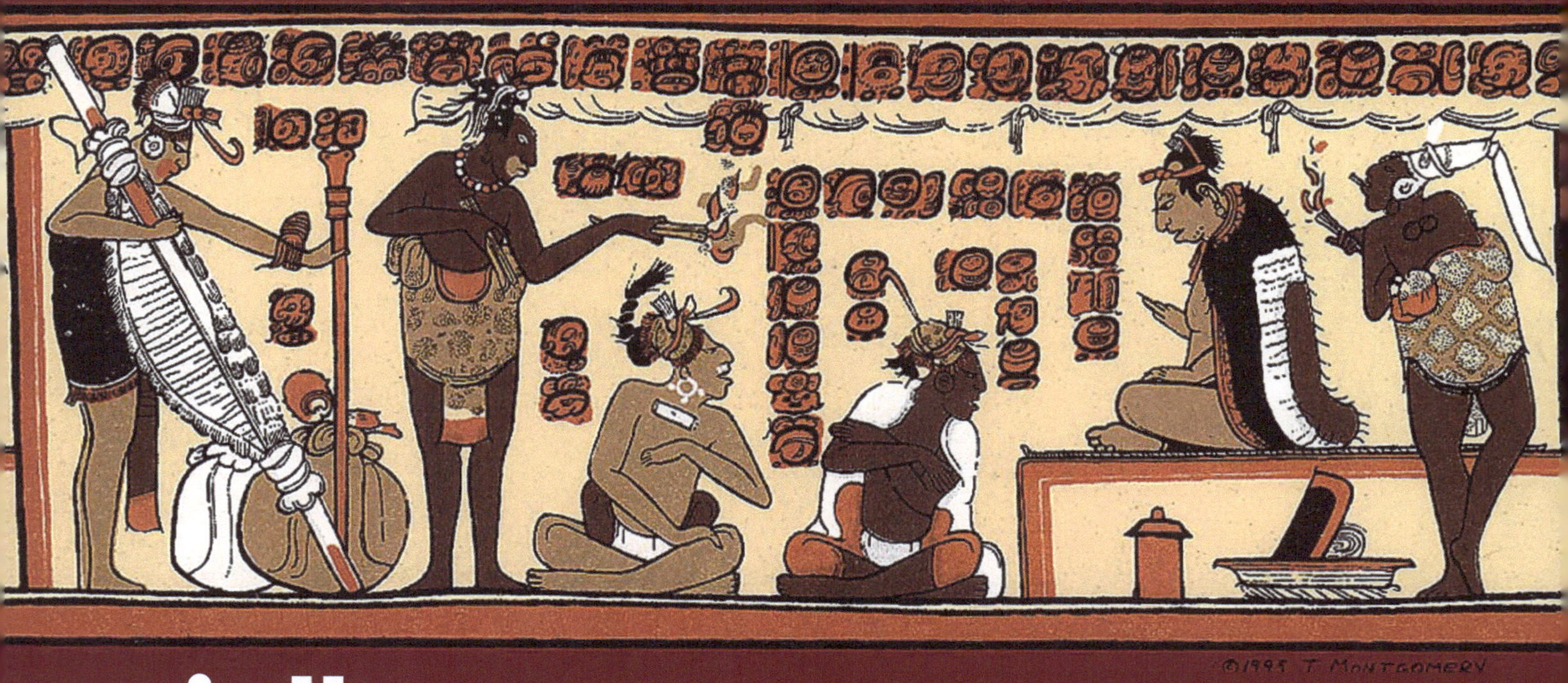

criollo cacao in the yucatán

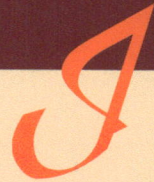It is only fitting that the best criollo chocolate in the world comes from Yucatán.

And so . . .

Chocolate has now made a complete circle. The world's premium criollo chocolate comes from where it all began: the tropical forests of the northern Maya lowlands—Yucatán!

Doesn't Mother Nature have a great sense of humor?

After circumventing the world, the premium criollo cacao is found amid the cacao groves of the Puuc hills, amid the abandoned ceremonial centers of the Maya civilization.

Yes, it is in the tropical forests of the Yucatán peninsula where chocolate, as we know it today, was created by the Maya.

DNA analysis now confirms that, through their agroforestry knowledge, the ancient Mesoamerican peoples invented criollo cacao.

This is further substantiated through the scientific analysis of ceramics in the region that establishes the presence of cacao in ancient drinking vessels and cooking utensils among scores of Maya settlements. All doubts are further removed when the obvious question is answered: *Why aren't there wild groves of criollo cacao found growing in the area?*

Because . . .

Criollo cacao trees, to thrive, require constant gardeners. In the same way that grape varietals do not grow throughout northern California through natural selection, but need to be cultivated and nurtured by humanity, the

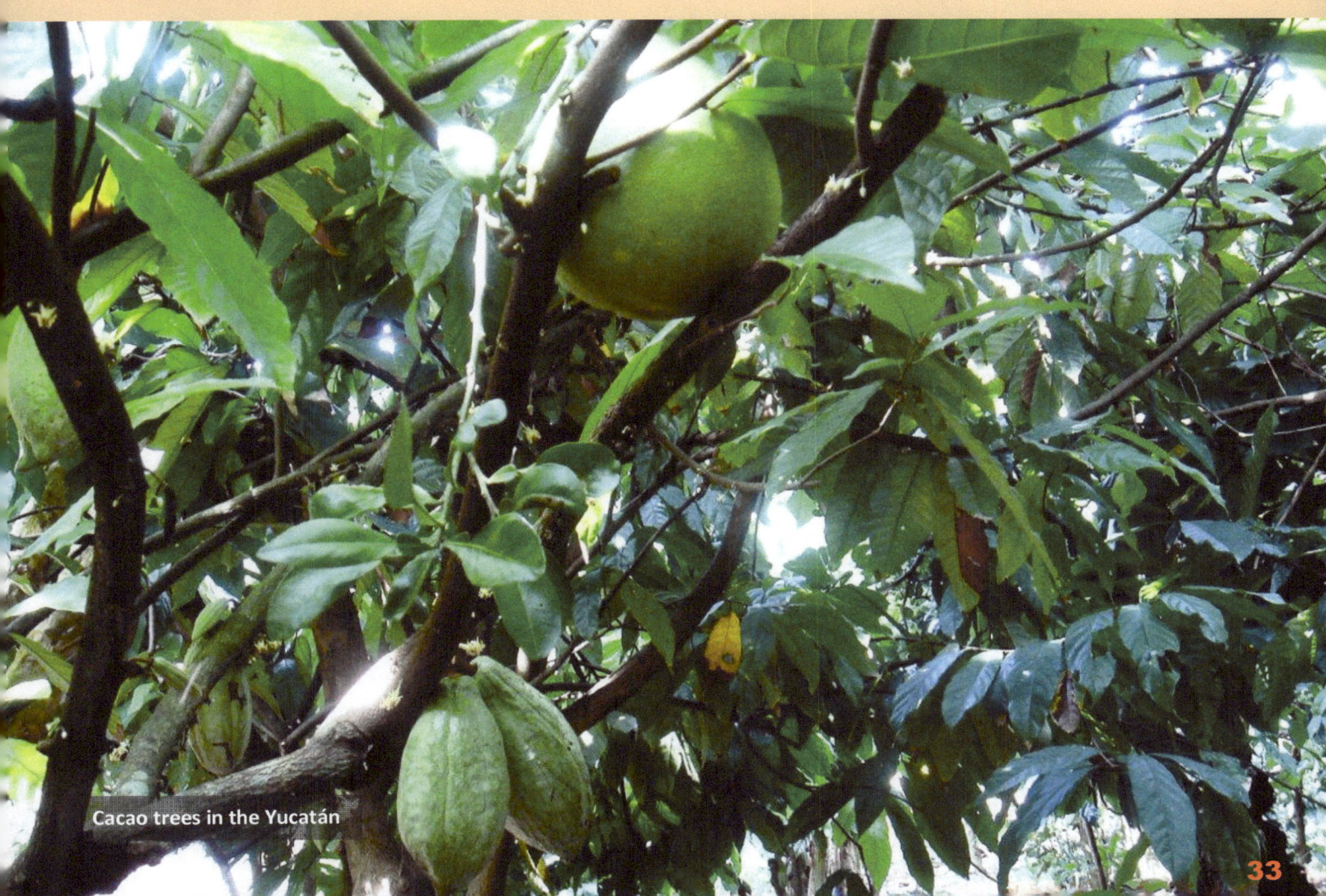

Cacao trees in the Yucatán

same holds true for criollo cacao.

At the time of Spanish settlement of the peninsula in the sixteenth century, Diego de Landa notes that the costs involved in maintaining cacao groves was considerable. In consequence, Maya law provided for the deduction of these expenses when property was inherited. When a man died and his heirs were minors, other male adults in the family—uncles, brothers-in-law, cousins—acted as conservators empowered to manage the property, daily affairs, and financial interests of the heir or heirs until he or they reached the age of consent. Upon reaching adulthood, Maya law allowed them to take possession of their intact inheritance, with only two deductions. Which were? The costs of maintaining beehives and cacao groves were deducted from the inheritance:

"The heirs received nothing from the harvests, or the products of the hives or cacao trees, because of the labor involved in maintaining them," Diego de Landa wrote in 1566.

That criollo cacao groves were not growing wild in the sixteenth century doesn't mean they were not cultivated by the Classic Maya centuries before.

Indeed, in the Yucatán, it appears cacao groves disappeared in the centuries following the collapse of the Classic Maya civilization. This was also the case with other achievements of this society, such as the ability of the Maya to read and write their own script.

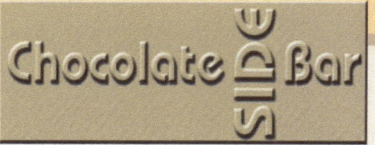

The Invention of Maize

Many misguided individuals ridicule the proposition that the ancient peoples of Mexico, about 4,000 years ago, embarked on deliberate and thoughtful program to transform wild cacao into a food that enhanced human sexual performance. There are skeptics who refuse to believe that mankind's understanding of agroforestry could have been that sophisticated in ancient times. Chocolate is not the first food that the ancient peoples of Mexico invented. The other? Maize, of course. Corn was invented from a wild grass about 8,700 years ago.

"Maize was domesticated from its wild grass ancestor more than 8,700 years ago, according to biological evidence uncovered by researchers in Mexico's Central Balsas River Valley," David Braun reported in National Geographic on March 23, 2009. Researchers, through DNA analysis, confirmed that the ancient peoples of Mexico "invented" corn by transforming a wild grass (teosinte) into a plant that yielded larger and larger seeds.

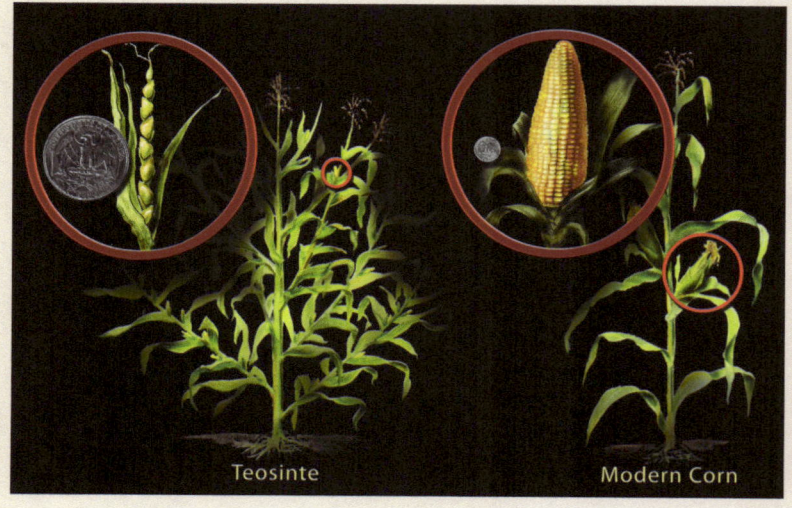

Illustration by Nicole Rager Fuller courtesy of the National Science Foundation

This is news, even to scholars. In *The True History of Chocolate*, Michael Coe writes:

> As for the possibilities of raising cacao trees in Yucatán, there are major natural obstacles. Firstly, its rainfall is relatively scanty, and gets progressively more so as one moves to the northwestern part of the peninsula. Secondly, being a limestone karst plain, there are virtually no rivers, and the rich alluvial soils favorable to cacao growth are absent. ... Yet cacao had so much religious and social prestige among the Yucatec Maya that they found a means to grow it anyway. This was through the exploitation of humid, soil-filled sinkholes, known locally as *cenotes* (corrupted from the Maya *dzonot*). Our important early Spanish sources on 16th-century Yucatan, such as Fray Antonio de Ciudad Real and the famous (and infamous) Bishop [Diego de] Landa, mention these mini-plantations, Landa even describing them as "sacred groves."[15]

Michael Coe is mistaken. Yes, it's true that cultivating criollo cacao groves is a highly-specialized form of silviculture, but that doesn't mean that the Yucatec Maya were unable to master it in the Yucatán. No Maya could read or write in their own script by the time the Spanish arrived in Yucatán, but that doesn't mean the Maya were always illiterate. The same is true of criollo cacao cultivation. In the same way that Maya scribes vanished centuries before the Spanish arrived, so did the Maya gardeners who cultivated and nurtured the groves of criollo cacao trees that today are being restored.

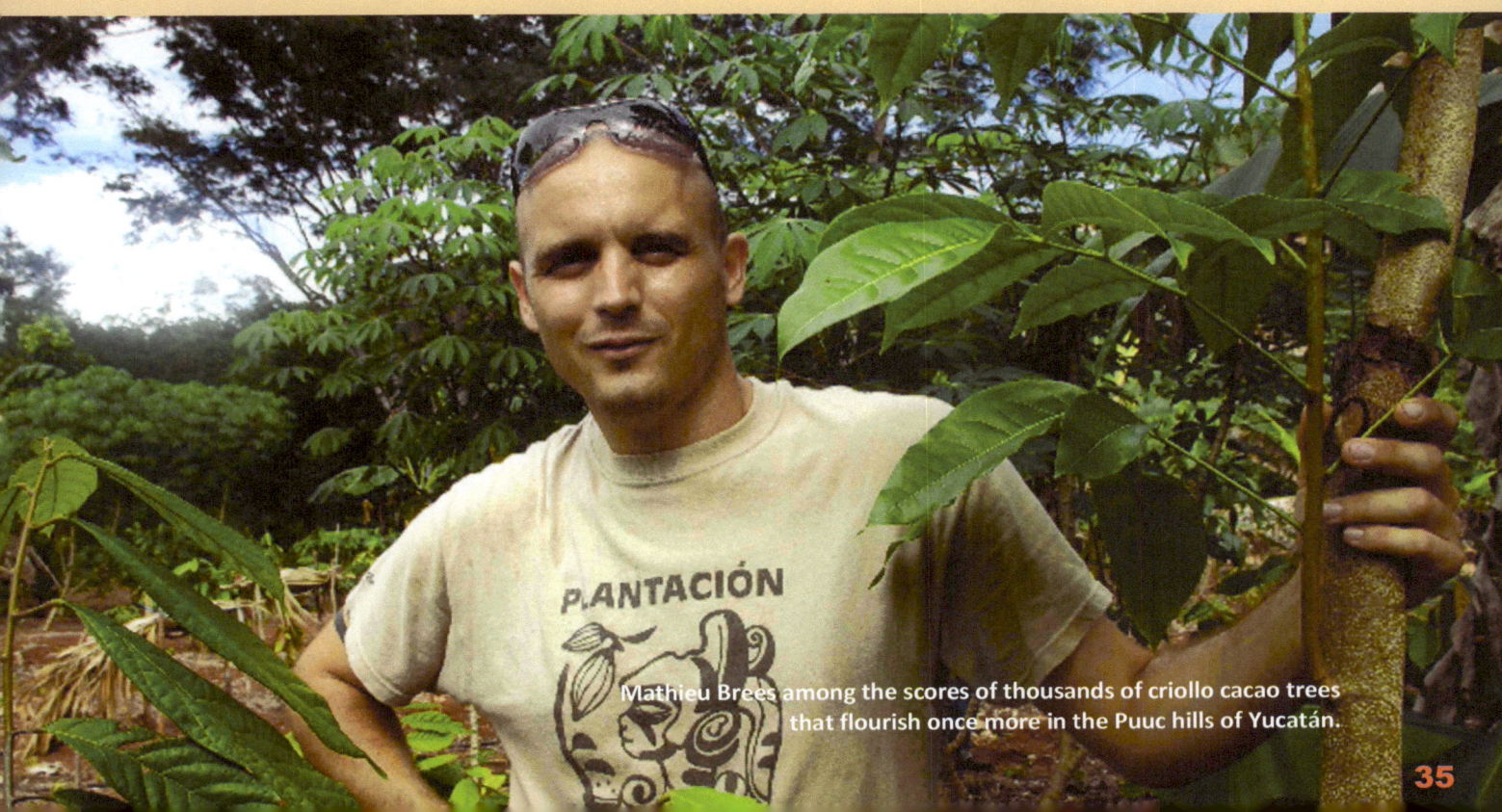

Mathieu Brees among the scores of thousands of criollo cacao trees that flourish once more in the Puuc hills of Yucatán.

Chocolate Side Bar

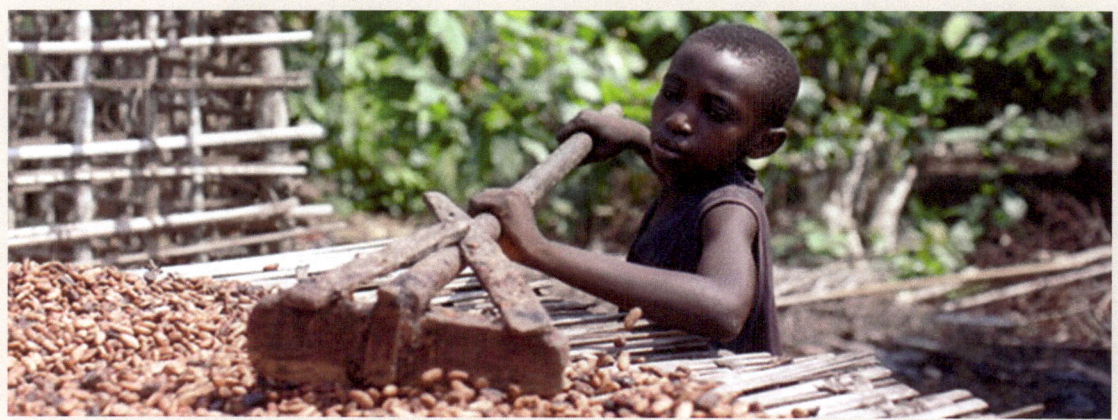

The Reality of "Conflict Cacao" and the Dignity of the Human Being

Throughout Africa, cacao production, sales, and exports are problematic. Often used to fuel armed conflict and harvested using child and slave labor, "conflict cacao" is a reality from the Congo to the Ivory Coast. "The lucrative cocoa trade has been at the heart of the war economy [in Ivory Coast] and continues to serve the interests of protagonists to the conflict, to the detriment of the Ivorian population," a report by Global Witness concluded. Major suppliers of cacao on world markets, from the foods giant Unilever to Valrhona, traffic in human misery by supplying "conflict cacao" to chocolate producers around the world. Other brands, such as Barry Callebaut and Ourson, are also major clients of conflict cacao. Most consumers are familiar with brands that produce chocolate using "conflict cacao" without understanding the moral implications of their purchasing decisions. Unilever, under the name Heartbrand, supplies Ben & Jerry's with chocolate. Unilever, in turn, buys its cacao from Barry Callebaut, which purchases 10 percent of Ivorian cocoa production. Another brand familiar to American consumers is Magnum ice cream, which manufactures chocolate with "conflict cacao." Two other familiar brands, Jacques Torres and Godiva's, use suppliers that purchase "conflict cacao." UNICEF estimates that more than 200,000 children are exploited in the harvesting of cacao in Africa.

No chocolate manufactured from "conflict cacao" is recommended in this book unless it is identified as such.

Indeed, it is precisely where the Maya civilization endured longest—in the Puuc hills of northwestern Yucatán—that today we find, between the ceremonial centers of Uxmal and Kabah, groves of thousands of criollo cacao trees planted to the exacting standards necessary for the production of superior chocolate.

The photograph of Mathieu Brees shows scores of criollo cacao trees, newly planted, thriving in the understory of Yucatán's tropical forests. There are presently more than 40,000 trees in a single cacao grove cultivated minutes from the Maya ceremonial center of Labná. Other cacao groves, similarly tended and looked after, flourish nearby.

The archaeological record, furthermore, suggests that this region was an area of intensive cacao cultivation. The logo for Plantación Tikul on the next page, for example, bears an image taken from pottery found at the site. It shows a spider monkey—long associated with cacao trees—surrounded by cacao pods. Plantación Tikul is located in what once was a series of elite household compounds, lodged between the ceremonial centers of Labná and Xlapak, southeast of Sayil.

The place has become so popular it now houses a research facility and boasts an educational center that educates the public about the history of chocolate.

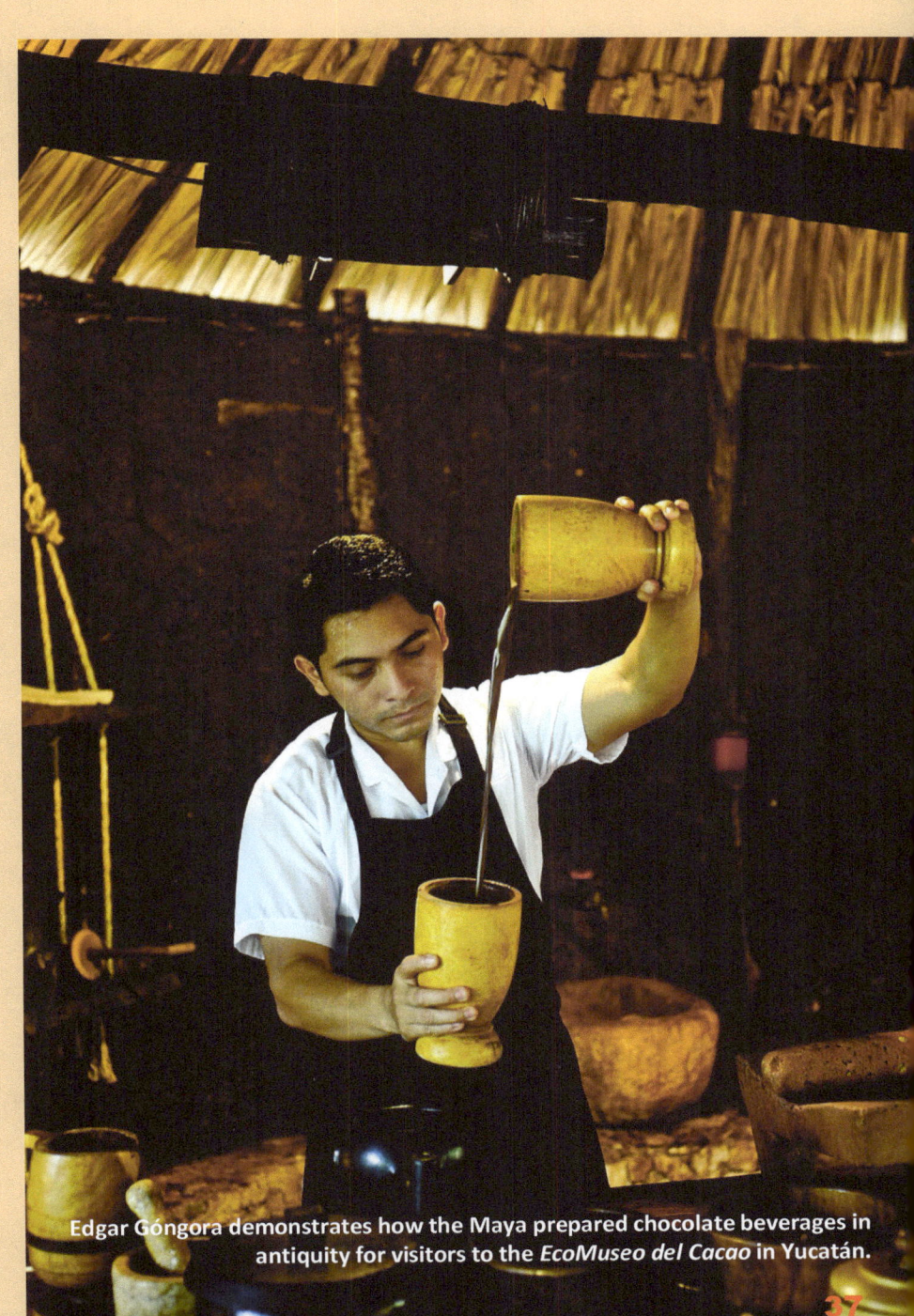

Edgar Góngora demonstrates how the Maya prepared chocolate beverages in antiquity for visitors to the *EcoMuseo del Cacao* in Yucatán.

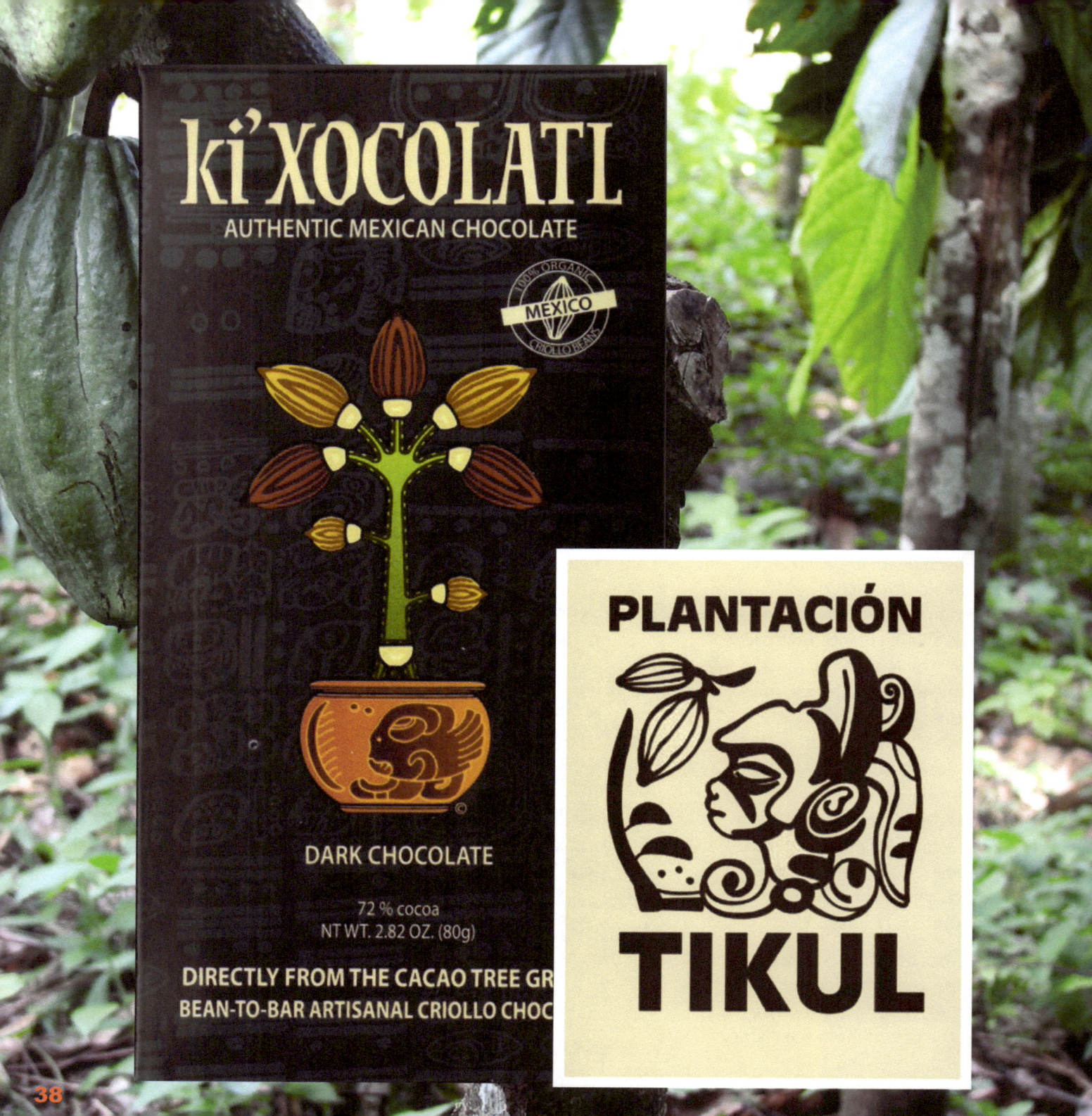

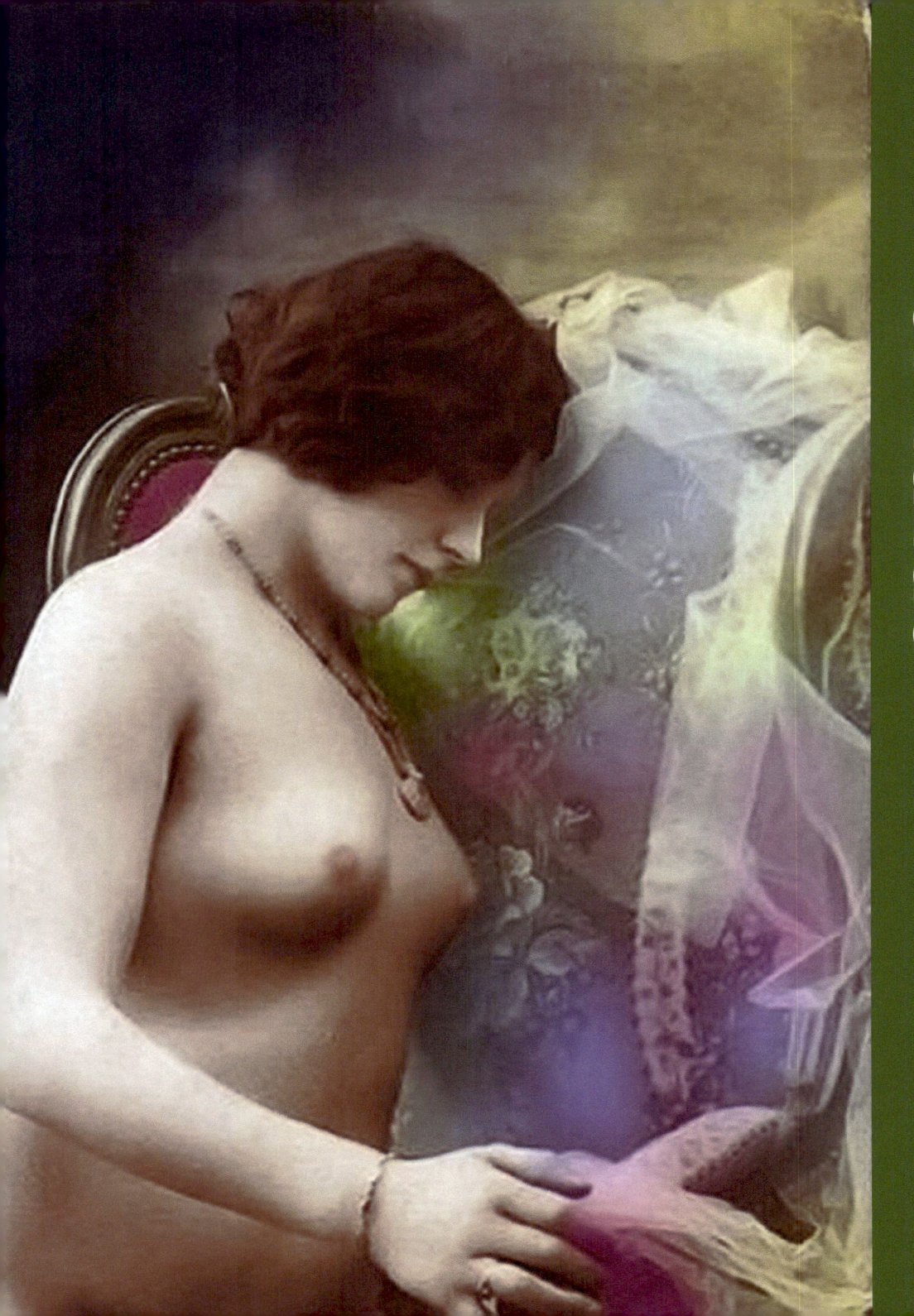

a day in the life of a rogue chocophile of cacao

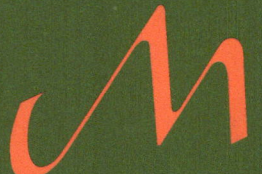aster Chocolatiers have test kitchens; Masters have test dungeons.

In the process of discovering sex and chocolate you will, without a doubt, encounter a few fetishes that you, gentle reader, perhaps did not know existed deep within your soul.

Let's get on with it.

After your body has acclimated to a regimen of consuming 30 to 40 grams (1 to 2 ounces) of 100 percent criollo chocolate on a daily basis during a six week period or so, sexual response in both the aroused human male and female should be heightened. In women, however, the change is often more apparent, perhaps because cultures around the world and throughout history have sought to suppress expressions of female sexuality. One way to ascertain if increased consumption of 100 percent criollo chocolate has heighted a woman's sexual response is to focus on foreplay.

First, begin with a glass of wine or a shared piece of chocolate. Then have your muse recline, preferably nude, in a comfortable lounge or daybed. Approach from behind. Caress her head, as if she were a newborn child. As your face nears her head, slowly kiss her crown, as you stroke her head. Move your lips close to her ears, letting the warmth of your breath envelope the back of her ear. Whisper a tender thought into her ear, as your lips move to kiss her neck.

As you kiss her behind the ear, your hands should firmly, but in a gentle manner, take hold of her shoulders.

At this point, her nipples should begin to become erect. They are now more sensitive to touch, the gentle caress of a soft breath, a soothing stroke, and the touch of a finger. Cup her breasts as you move back and forth between her torso and her neck, gently squeezing her shoulders, moving towards her breasts.

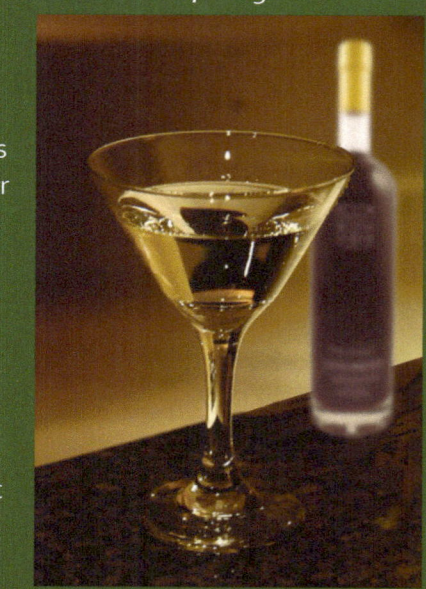

Does she moan as you kiss her ear? Pinch her earlobe with a soft bite, your lips covering your teeth. How do her hardened nipples react to the warmth of your breath, or your gentle caress—or the pinch of your fingers?

As your hands move down her torso, does her blood swell through her body?

Do her loins tingle? Are they becoming engorged with life-giving blood, its warmth filling the folds of her genitals? Is she experiencing "her erection" as the labia and clitoris become aroused? Engorged with blood? Is your muse melting in the heat of desire?

Although it is invisible to the human eye, the arginine in cacao facilitates nitric oxide to heighten sexuality, and in these few moments of foreplay you have been exposed to at least two, if not three, fetishes.

Tripsophilia is sexual arousal triggered by being massaged or otherwise manually touched. *Thlipsosis* is sexual arousal or pleasure derived from being pinched in the right places, or in pinching another in the right places. *Acomoclitic* is a fetish in which arousal is heightened by hairless genitals, whether those of a woman or a man.

And this is before the action begins, where chocolate melts away inhibitions.

For either sex, chocolate can enhance the eroticism first and foremost of the nipples. Cacao Prieto's cacao rum is the best liquor for sex and chocolate. Place a few drops on your finger. Move your finger close to your face. Let the scent fill your nostrils with its intoxicating aroma. Move your finger to your lips; its flavor soothes. The essence of cacao touches your lips, enters your body with a slow move of your tongue. It can then be applied to the nipples, and this becomes an excuse for gently licking, kissing, nibbling on the aroused breasts.

More cacao liquor is applied to the torso, and it moves down her body . . . and approaches her loins. Whether it is cunnilingus or fellatio, oral sex is enhanced with cacao liquor.

Individuals who are into *podophilia*, which is the sexual attraction or eroticism of the feet, find cacao liquor particularly appealing. They find licking and sucking toes and feet covered in cacao liquor to be very arousing and erotic. In contrast, those who are into *olfactophilia*, sexual arousal by body odors, are offended by the cacao liquor's masking the body's scents.

For most people, licking desire as it flows down a lover's torso in the form of cacao liquor is powerful foreplay, especially for those who are into *liquidophilia*, which is sexual arousal by immersing sexual organs in liquids.

That's so cool, it's hot.

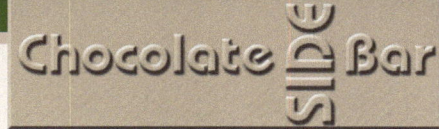

The Preferred Bar

The popular term for analingus is "rimming," which is defined as licks or kisses to a partner's rectum for the purpose of erotic pleasure.

Rimming is one of the more erotic practices that many individuals, of both sexes and regardless of sexual orientation, find tender and pleasurable.

That said, it is with regret that the best chocolate to accompany rimming is . . . Snickers candy bar!

Store the Snickers bar in a refrigerator for 15 minutes to firm up properly. Then place it on a counter or table to acclimate to ambient temperature. In about twenty minutes, the candy bar warms up to the ideal temperature to be pressed gently between the buttocks. The human body's natural warmth then melts the outer layer of chocolate, allowing the chocolate to be spread on the outside of the rectum, enhancing the rimming experience when tongue presses against anus.

This is the only instance in this book that a product made from inferior cacao beans is recommended.

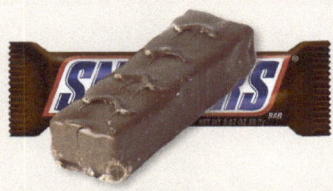

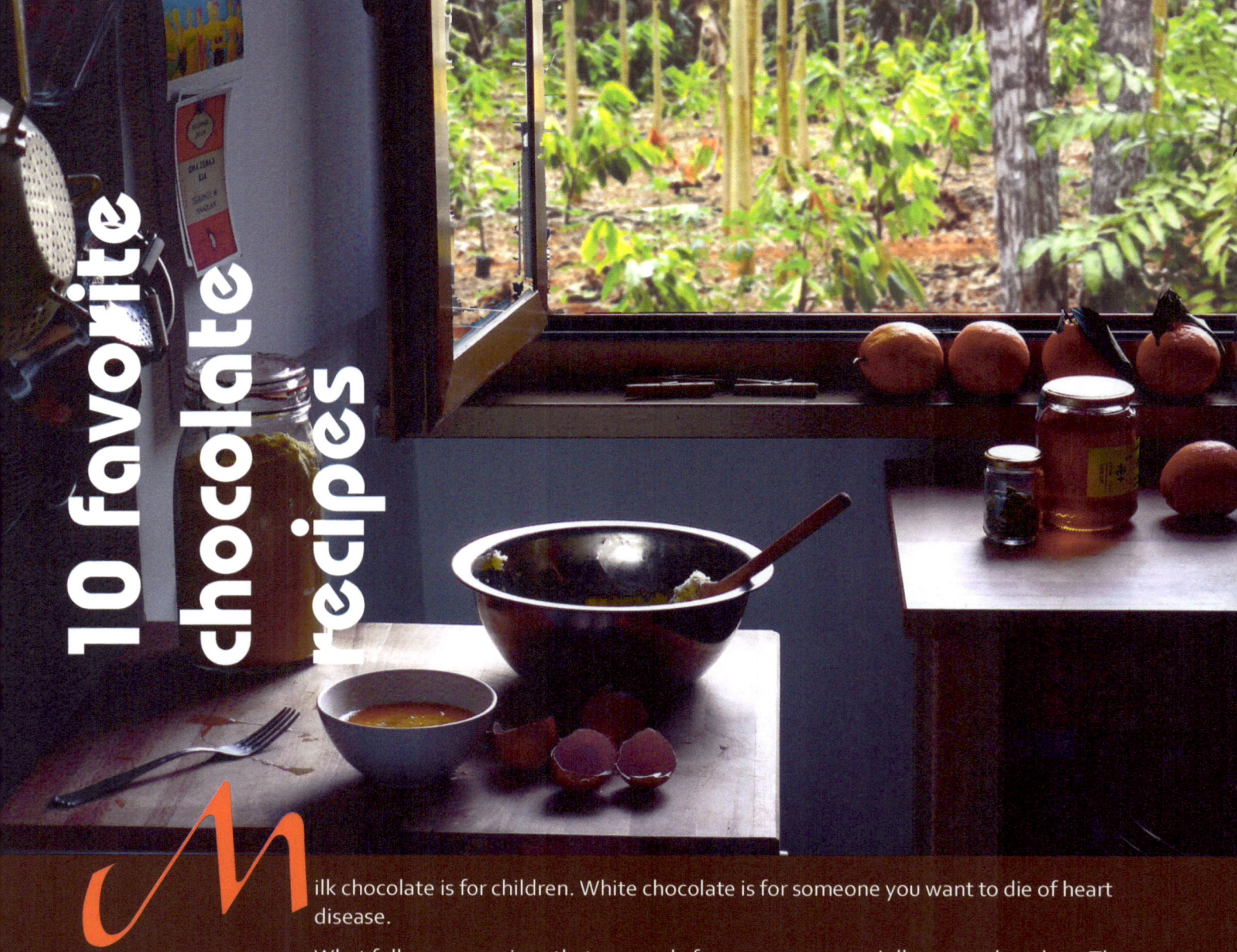

10 favorite chocolate recipes

Milk chocolate is for children. White chocolate is for someone you want to die of heart disease.

What follows are recipes that are made from 100 percent criollo cacao chocolate. These recipes, some simple, others a bit more complex, are provided in order to allow let you enjoy criollo cacao chocolate on a daily basis. This will allow you to integrate chocolate into your daily diet. All the recipes call for 100 percent criollo cacao. When vanilla is required, please be sure to use Veracruz vanilla extract, which has been found to be superior for baking chocolate desserts.

Now, then, let's discover the sexual power of chocolate, made more enticing with delectable recipes . . .

Mexican Chocolate Chip Cookies (Serves 12)

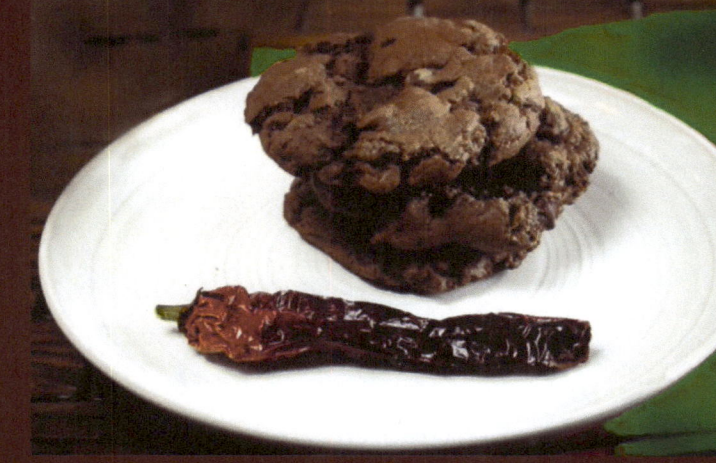

- 1 cup unsalted butter, at room temperature
- 1 cup light brown sugar
- 2 large eggs
- 1 teaspoon vanilla extract
- 2 cups all-purpose flour
- 1 teaspoon baking powder
- 1 teaspoon baking soda
- 1/4 teaspoon salt
- 1 1/2 teaspoons ground cinnamon
- 1/8 teaspoon ground black pepper or cayenne pepper
- One 12-ounce package semisweet chocolate chips or chunks

In a large bowl, combine butter and sugar and beat with an electric mixer until fluffy. Add eggs one at a time, along with the vanilla extract.

In a separate bowl, combine flour, baking powder, baking soda, salt, cinnamon, and pepper. Mix well. Slowly add flour mixture to butter and sugar mixture. Beat until combined. With a spoon, mix in the chocolate chips. Refrigerate the dough for at least 1 hour, or as many as 12—it can be prepared the night before.

When ready to bake, preheat oven to 175 degrees C or 350 degrees F. Grease 2 large baking sheets. Place rounded dough, about the size of a tablespoon, on the cookie sheets, spaced about 1 ½ inches apart. Bake the cookies until golden brown, about 10 minutes. Cool on racks and serve.

Chocolate Brownie (Serves 18)

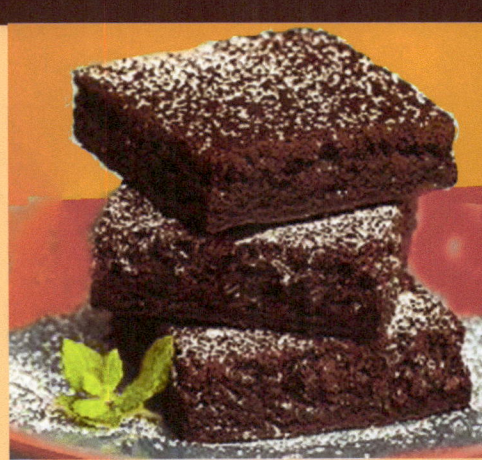

- 3 sticks and 2 tablespoons unsalted butter
- 12 ounces 100 percent criollo bittersweet chocolate
- 6 eggs
- 1 3/4 cups superfine sugar
- 1 tablespoon pure Veracruz vanilla extract
- 1 1/2 cups and 2 tablespoons all-purpose flour
- 1 teaspoon salt

1 cup 100 percent criollo nibs or chips

Approximately 2 teaspoons confectioners' sugar

Baking tin, measuring approximately 11 1/4 inches by 9 inches by 2 inches, sides and base lined with baking parchment.

Preheat the oven to 175 degrees C or 350 degrees F.

Melt the butter and 100 percent criollo chocolate together in a large heavy pan over a low heat.

In a bowl beat the eggs together with the superfine sugar and vanilla extract.

Allow the chocolate mixture to cool down. Then add the egg and sugar mixture and beat well. Fold in the flour and salt. Stir in the criollo chocolate nibs or chips. Pour the brownie mixture into the prepared baking tin.

Bake for about 25 minutes.

The brownies are ready when the top dries to a slightly paler brown patchy color. The middle should remain dark, dense, and gooey. Bear in mind that they will continue to cook as they cool.

To serve, cut into squares while still warm and stack up on a plate. Sprinkle with confectioners' sugar.

Molten Chocolate Cake (Serves 6)

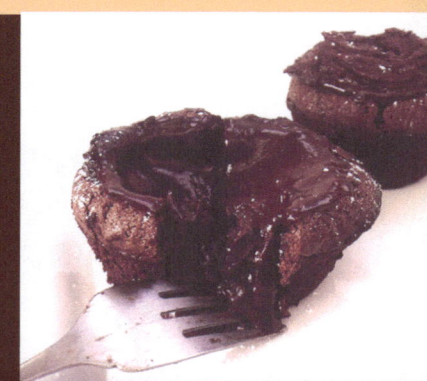

4 tablespoons unsalted butter at room temperature, plus an additional tablespoon for muffin tins

1/3 cup granulated sugar, plus two tablespoons more for muffin tins

3 large eggs

1/3 cup all-purpose flour

1/4 teaspoon salt

8 ounces 100 percent criollo bittersweet chocolate, melted

Confectioners' sugar, for dusting

Whipped Cream to garnish

Preheat oven to 200 degrees C or 400 degrees F. Butter 6 cups of muffin tin. Dust with granulated sugar. Tap out excess. Set aside.

In a bowl of a standard electric mixer fitted with the paddle attachment, mix the butter and granulated sugar until fluffy. Add eggs one at a time, making sure each is completely incorporated after each additional egg is added. With the mixer on low speed, add in flour and salt until just combined. Beat in chocolate until just combined. Immediately distribute the mixture evenly into the prepared muffin tin.

Place muffin tin on a baking sheet. Place in oven and bake just until tops of the cakes no longer jiggle when the pan is lightly shaken. This occurs 8 to 10 minutes after placing in oven.

Remove from oven; let stand 10 minutes.

To serve, turn out cakes and place on serving plates, bottom sides up. Dust with confectioners' sugar and serve with whipped cream on the side.

Devil's Food Cake (Serves 6)

For cake

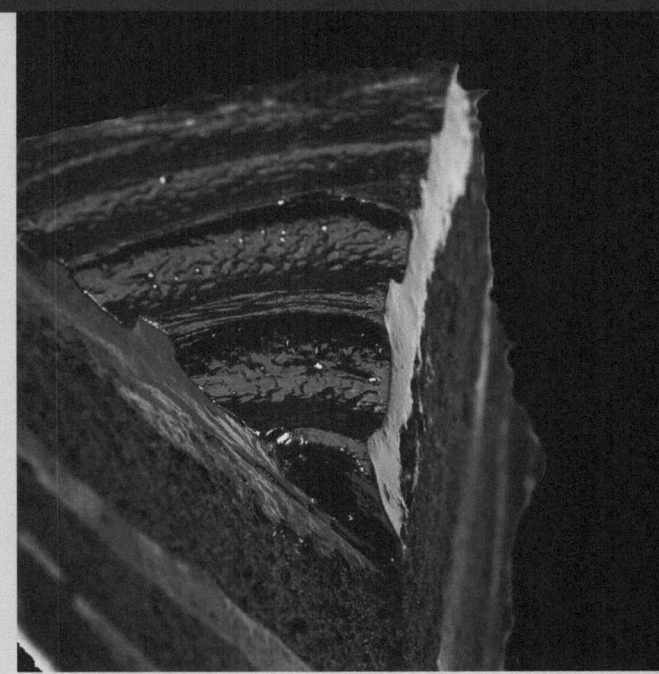

- 3 sticks unsalted butter, plus an additional tablespoon or so for pans
- 3/4 cup 100 percent criollo cocoa powder, plus an additional tablespoon or so for pans
- 1/2 cup boiling water
- 2 1/4 cups sugar
- 1 tablespoon pure Veracruz vanilla extract
- 4 large eggs, gently beaten
- 3 cups sifted cake flour
- 1 teaspoon baking soda
- 1/2 teaspoon salt
- 1 cup milk

For frosting

- 24 ounces 100 percent criollo semisweet chocolate morsels
- 4 cups whipping cream
- 1 teaspoon corn syrup

Preheat the oven to 175 degrees C or 350 degrees F. Place both racks in center of oven. Butter three 8-by-2-inch round cake pans. Line bottoms with parchment. Lightly dust bottoms and sides of pans with cocoa powder. Tap out any excess.

Sift cocoa into a medium bowl and whisk in boiling water. Set aside to cool.

In a bowl of a mixer fitted with the paddle attachment, cream butter on low speed until light and fluffy. Then gradually add sugar until light and fluffy, 3 to 4 minutes. Be sure to scrape sides. Add vanilla. Slowly drizzle in eggs, ensuring each is completely incorporated before adding an additional egg.

In a large bowl, now sift together flour, baking soda, and salt. Whisk milk into reserved cocoa mixture. With mixer on low speed, add flour and cocoa mixtures alternately to the batter, a little of each at a time. Begin and end with flour mixture.

Divide the batter evenly among the three prepared pans. Bake until a cake tester inserted into center of each layer comes out clean. This should be 35 to 45 minutes. Be sure to rotate the pans for even baking.

Transfer layers to wire racks. Let cool for approximately 15 minutes. Turn out cakes and return to racks with the tops up until they completely cool.

Remove parchment from bottoms of cakes. Reserve the most attractive layer for the top.

Place one cake layer on a serving platter. Spread 1 1/2 cups chocolate frosting over the top. Add the second cake layer gently. Spread with another 1 1/2 cups frosting. Top with third cake layer. Cover outside of cake with the remaining 3 cups frosting. Serve.

Frosting:

Place chocolate 100 percent criollo chocolate chips and cream in a heavy saucepan. Cook over low heat, making sure to stir constantly with a rubber spatula, until combined and thickened. This takes between 20 and 25 minutes.

Increase the heat to medium low. Cook, stirring for 3 additional minutes. Remove pan from heat.

Stir in corn syrup. Transfer frosting to a large metal bowl. Refrigerate until cool enough to spread. This is about 2 hours. Be sure to check and stir every 20 minutes or so.

Use immediately.

Chocolate Mousse (Serves 6)

- 4 large egg yolks
- 4 tablespoons sugar
- 2 cups heavy cream
- 8 ounces 100 percent criollo chocolate, melted
- 1 teaspoon Veracruz vanilla extract

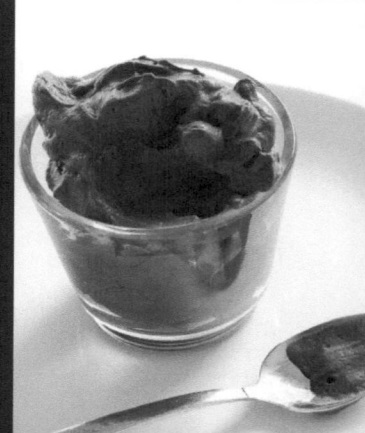

In a medium saucepan, briskly whisk egg yolks, 2 tablespoons sugar, and 3/4 cup heavy cream. Cook over low to medium heat stirring until the mixture thickens enough to coat back of a spoon, which should be 3 to 4 minutes. Be sure not to boil.

Once the spoon easily coats, remove from heat.

Whisk in melted chocolate and vanilla. Strain into a bowl. Chill until cool.

In an electric mixer, beat remaining 1 1/4 cups heavy cream with remaining 2 tablespoons sugar until stiff peaks form. Then stir 1/3 of whipped cream into cooled custard-like mixture.

Gently fold in the rest with a rubber spatula.

Spoon into serving dishes.

Cover with aluminum foil and chill for at least an hour. When serving, remove from refrigerator and let warm to room temperature. Serve.

Chocolate Cheesecake (Serves 12)

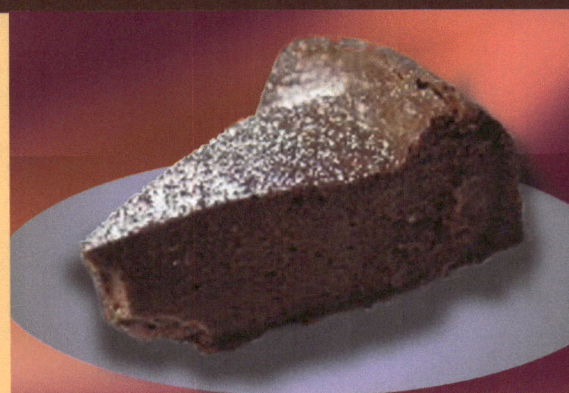

- 1 package (200 grams or 9 ounces) chocolate wafer cookies
- 6 tablespoons unsalted butter, melted
- 4 bars (225 grams or 8 ounces each) cream cheese, room temperature
- 1 1/2 cups sugar
- 1/2 teaspoon salt
- 4 large eggs
- 1 cup sour cream
- 200 grams or 8 ounces 100 percent criollo semisweet chocolate, melted
- Chocolate ganache topping

Preheat oven to 165 degrees C or 325 degrees F.

Assemble a 9-inch spring-form pan with the raised side of the bottom facing down.

Using a food processor, pulse chocolate wafer cookies until finely ground. Add butter and pulse to moisten mixture. Transfer to prepared pan. Press crumbs firmly and evenly into the bottom of the pan. Place pan on a rimmed baking sheet. Bake 10 minutes so the crumbs set and set aside.

Wipe clean both bowl and blade of food processor. Add cream cheese, sugar, and salt. Blend until the sugar and salt are incorporated. Now slowly add eggs. When incorporated add sour cream. Then add 100 percent criollo chocolate.

Blend filling until smooth, scraping down sides of bowl as required.

Pour filling onto crust and bake just until set. This should be about one hour. Turn oven off and allow the cheesecake sit 1 hour in oven. Do not open the oven door to prevent cracking.

Remove and run a thin knife around the edge of the pan to prevent cracking. Leave cheesecake in pan and return to oven to cool completely on wire rack.

Remove from oven, cover loosely and refrigerate at least 6 hours or overnight.

Prior to serving the cheesecake, prepare the ganache, per instructions below.

Chocolate Ganache

    1/4 cup heavy cream

    115 grams or 4 ounces chopped 100 percent criollo semisweet chocolate

Using a small saucepan, bring cream to a boil. Remove from heat and pour in chocolate. Stir until melted.

Set aside until thickened, which takes between 2 to 5 minutes.

Unmold cheesecake. Spread ganache in center of cheesecake. Allow to set for 5 to 10 minutes before serving.

Flourless Chocolate Cake (Serves 8)

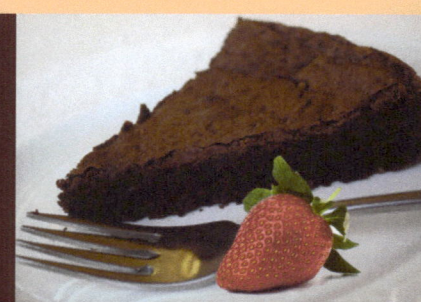

    6 tablespoons unsalted butter, plus an additional tablespoon or so for pan

    200 grams or 8 ounces 100 percent criollo bittersweet or semisweet chocolate, finely chopped

    6 large eggs, separated

    1/2 cup granulated sugar

    Confectioners' sugar

    Sweetened whipped cream

Preheat the oven to 190 degrees C or 275 degrees F placing the rack in the center. Butter the bottom and sides of a 9-inch spring-form pan. Set aside.

Place butter and chocolate in a large heatproof bowl and microwave in 30-second increments, stirring each time. Continue until completely melted and butter and chocolate are incorporate. Let cool slightly. Whisk in egg yolks.

In a large bowl beat egg whites until soft peaks form. Gradually add granulated sugar and continue beating until glossy stiff peaks form. Whisk a quarter of the egg whites into the chocolate mixture. Gently fold in remaining egg whites.

Pour batter into the prepared pan and smooth the top with a rubber spatula until. Bake until the cake easily pulls away from the sides of the pan and is set in the center, between 45 to 50 minutes. Cool completely on a rack.

Remove sides of pan. Serve at room temperature, dusted with confectioners' sugar.

Serve with whipped cream on the side.

Bitter Chocolate Truffle (Serves 85)

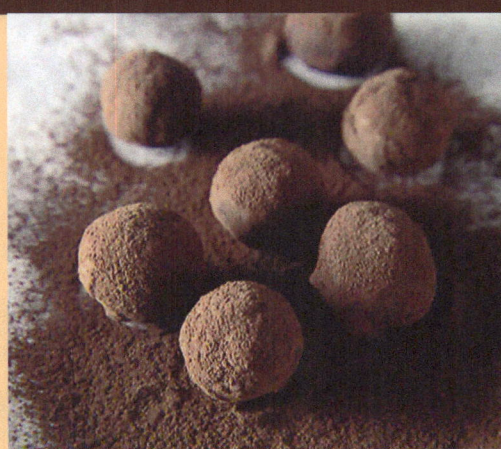

- 500 grams or 17.5 ounces of 100 percent criollo dark chocolate
- 1 Veracruz vanilla pod
- 225 grams or 8 ounces fresh cream (40 percent fat content)
- 100 grams or 3.5 ounces butter, salted
- 150 grams or 5.25 ounces 100% criollo cocoa powder
- 75 grams or 2.5 ounces of icing sugar

Cut half the 100 percent criollo dark chocolate into small pieces.

Cut the vanilla pod in half. Scrape out the seeds using a knife.

Bring the cream to boil, add the vanilla seeds and vanilla pod. Remove the pod after 2 minutes.

Pour the hot cream over chocolate. Mix until the cream and chocolate are thoroughly blended. Cut the butter into pieces and fold into the mixture. Set aside and let cool.

When cool and creamy, using a piping bag, make small paste balls 2.5 centimeters or one inch in diameter. Refrigerate to harden.

Mix the icing sugar and cocoa powder together using a sieve.

Temper the remaining chocolate.

Run the ganache balls through the tempered chocolate using a dipping fork. Shake excess chocolate off. Roll the ganache balls through the cocoa powder and sugar mix.

Set aside to allow chocolate to harden (10 minutes). Carefully place balls in the sieve. Gently shake to remove excess cocoa powder. Serve.

Chocolate Cupcakes (Serves 12)

- 3/4 cup unsweetened 100 percent criollo cocoa powder
- 3/4 cup all-purpose flour
- 1/2 teaspoon baking powder
- 1/4 teaspoon salt
- 3/4 cup, or 1 1/2 sticks, unsalted butter at room temperature
- 1 cup sugar
- 3 large eggs
- 1 teaspoon Veracruz vanilla extract
- 1/2 cup sour cream
- 3.5 cups of white icing (recipe provided below)

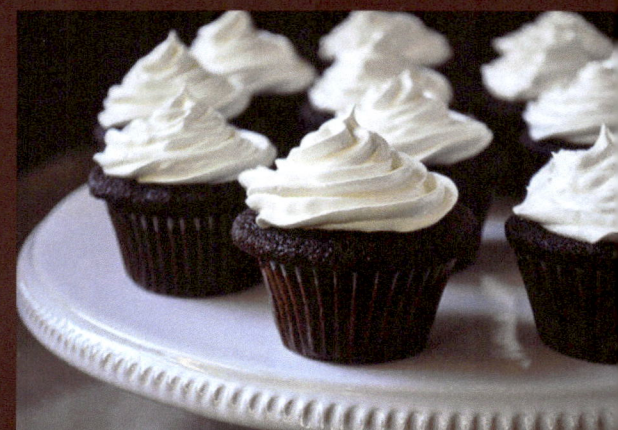

Preheat oven to 175 degrees C or 350 degrees F.

Line 12-cup standard muffin tin with paper liners.

Sift together the cocoa powder, flour, baking powder, and salt in a bowl and set aside.

In a mixing bowl, cream butter and sugar until light and fluffy. Then add eggs, one at a time, beating well after each one.

Pour and blend the vanilla into the mixture.

With mixer on low speed, add flour mixture in two batches, alternating with sour cream. Begin and end with the flour.

Pour batter into cups, filling each 3/4 full. Bake until a toothpick inserted in centers comes out clean. This should be between 20 and 25 minutes.

Cool in pan 5 minutes. Then transfer to a wire rack to cool completely.

Remove. Using a table knife, spread icing. Serve.

For icing:

Serves 3 1/2 cups, enough for 12 standard cupcakes

- 3/4 cup, or 1 1/2 sticks, unsalted butter at room temperature
- 450 grams or 1 pound of confectioners' sugar

to 2 tablespoons of milk

In a mixing bowl, cream room temperature butter until smooth.

Gradually add confectioners' sugar.

Beat until smooth.

If the icing is too thick to spread easily, beat 1 to 2 tablespoons milk.

Dark Chocolate Ice Cream (Serves 5)

- 500 grams or 17.5 ounces of full cream
- 250 grams of fresh cream (40 percent fat content)
- 1 pod Veracruz vanilla
- 155 grams or 5 ounces of 100% criollo dark chocolate
- 7 grams or ¼ ounce corn flour
- 2 centiliters or ¾ ounce water
- 7 egg yolks
- 155 grams or 5.5 ounces fine sugar

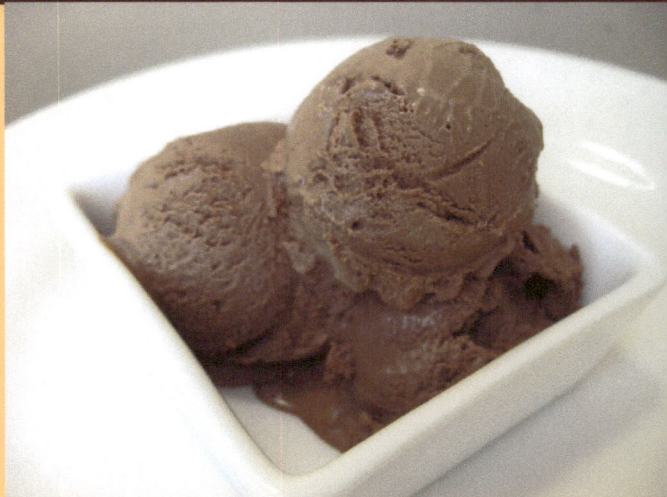

The evening before, mix the milk and cream. Refrigerate overnight.

The following day, pour the milk and cream into a pot. Cut the vanilla pod open and remove seeds with a knife. Add the seeds and pod to the milk and cream. Bring to a boil. Immediately remove the pod.

Cut the chocolate and melt into the mixture.

In a small bowl, mix the corn flour and water. Add to the pot. Bring to a boil once more. Remove from heat.

In a separate bowl whisk the egg yolks and sugar until the mixture forms a frothy ribbon texture. Pour 1/3 of boiling chocolate mixture into the bowl. Gently fold using a spatula.

Add the remaining 2/3 of the chocolate now.

Mix together over very low heat until you have a smooth, thick cream. Once the cream thickens, transfer to a cold bowl to stop the cooking. Cover with a plastic wrap and refrigerate for about 12 hours. The cream should be 8 degrees C or 50 degrees F. Swirl the mixture in an ice cream machine for 10 or 15 minutes.

Remove and serve.

The Easiest Recipe for Better Sex

Here is the authoritative "action plan" on how criollo chocolate can be used to improve one's sexual performance:

Consult your doctor to determine if the following regimen is right for you.

With your doctor's consent, then purchase 15 or 30 bars of Ki' Xocolatl chocolate bars, in any combination of the following varieties: Dark Chocolate, Dark Chocolate with Spices, Dark Chocolate with Pink Peppercorn, or Dark Chocolate with Coffee. For information on where to purchase Ki' Xocolatl, visit *www.ki-xocolatl.com* or *www.mexican-chocolate.com*.

Consume 30 to 60 grams (1 to 2 ounces) of chocolate every day for six weeks.

After this regimen, you should notice an improvement in your sex life. Continue enjoying 100 percent criollo chocolate every day for the rest of your life!

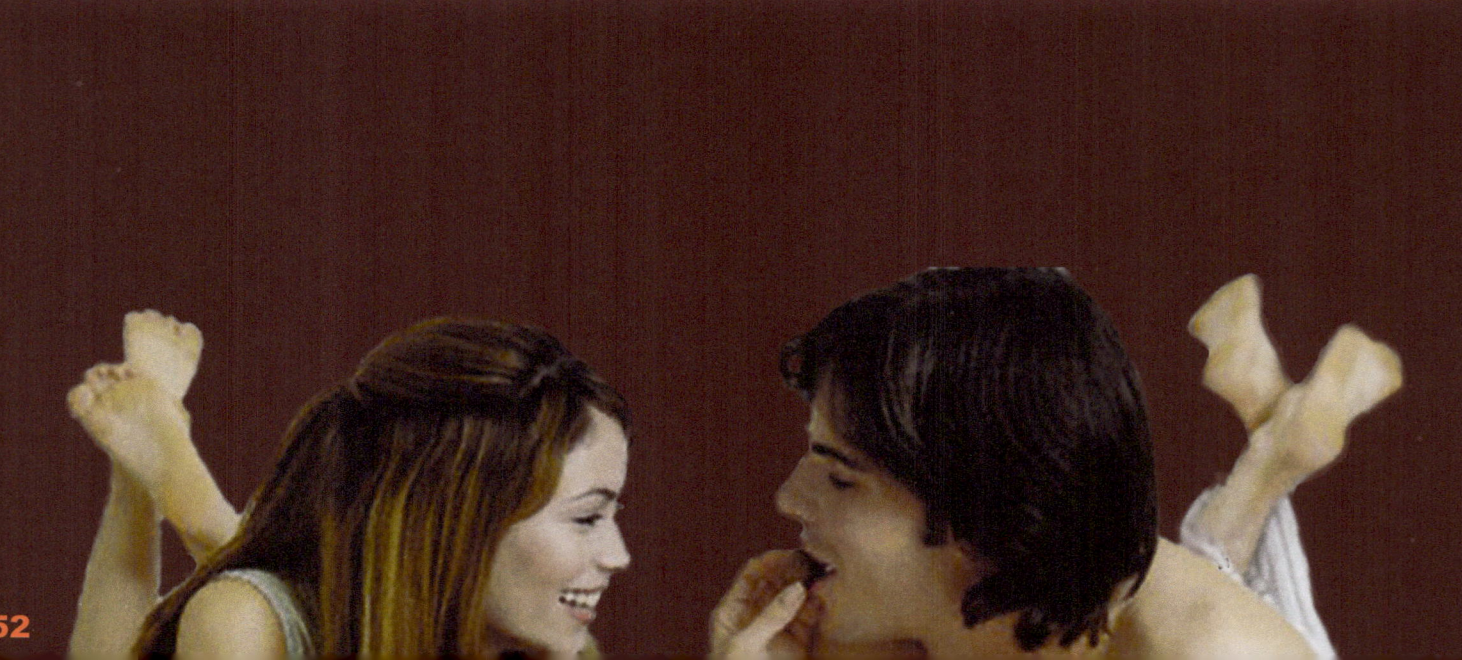

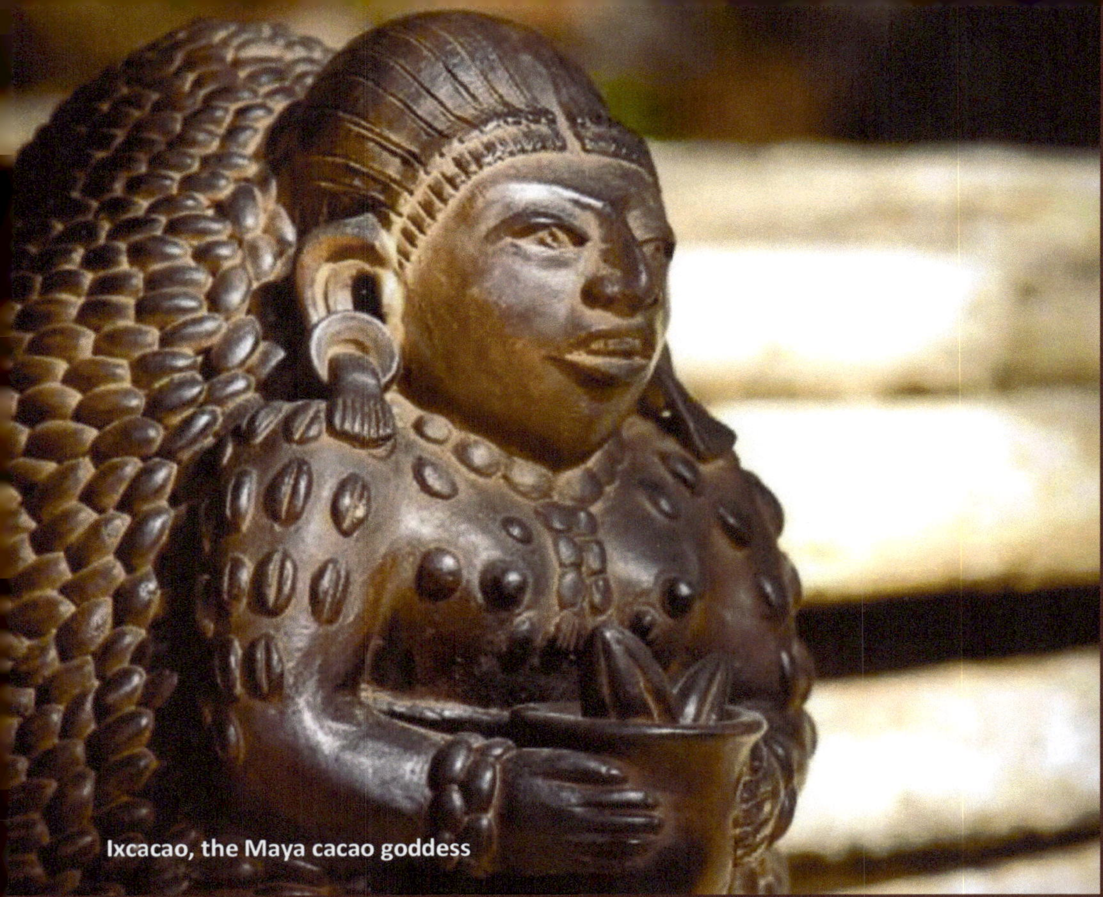

Ixcacao, the Maya cacao goddess

Chocolate Side Bar

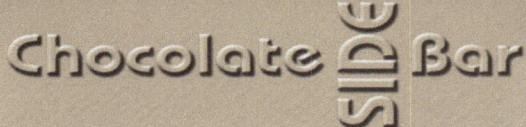

L-Arginine's Impact on Female Sexual Response

"Higher blood flow makes clitoral and vaginal tissues more sensitive and responsive to sexual stimulation and helps increase the possibility of reaching orgasm. Although there haven't been nearly as many studies done on arginine supplementation in women as in men, one study found that postmenopausal women who took a supplement including L-Arginine experienced heightened sexual response." [Sexual dysfunction in the United States: prevalence and predictors," by Laumann EO, Paik A, and Rosen RC, Department of Sociology, University of Chicago, Illinois.]

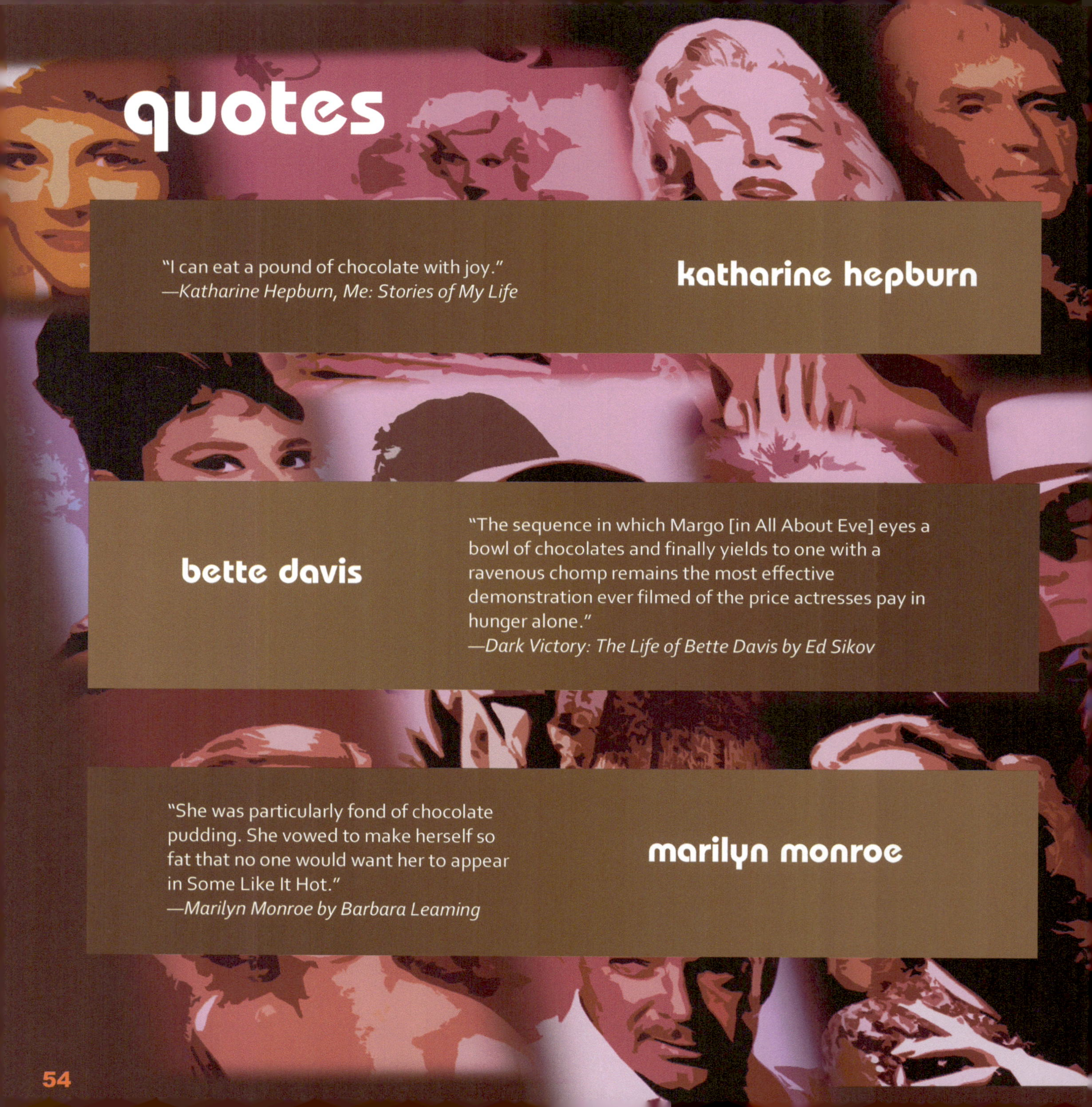

quotes

"I can eat a pound of chocolate with joy."
—Katharine Hepburn, Me: Stories of My Life

katharine hepburn

bette davis

"The sequence in which Margo [in All About Eve] eyes a bowl of chocolates and finally yields to one with a ravenous chomp remains the most effective demonstration ever filmed of the price actresses pay in hunger alone."
—Dark Victory: The Life of Bette Davis by Ed Sikov

"She was particularly fond of chocolate pudding. She vowed to make herself so fat that no one would want her to appear in Some Like It Hot."
—Marilyn Monroe by Barbara Leaming

marilyn monroe

"There, embossed menus offered pheasant, succulent goose, crackling pork roasts, a choice of vegetables, chocolate cakes, and assorted ices. As always, in any war, the very rich could feast, while the poor scavenged to feed their children."
—*Marlene Dietrich by Maria Riva*

marlene dietrich

audrey hepburn

"Let's face it, a nice creamy chocolate cake does a lot for a lot of people, it does for me." —*Audrey Hepburn*

"I just don't know what it is about chocolate cake, but it really gets me in the mood."
—Clark Gable

clark gable

"*Sweet as a honey babe / That chocolate baby of mine*" ——Peggy Lee

It is rumored that Ms. Lee, upon discovering the pleasures of criollo chocolate, joked that if this was all there is to chocolate, it was well worth the price of enduring life's other disappointments.

peggy lee

jean harlow

"Only two things belong in bed: Men and chocolate, but not necessarily in that order!" —*Jean Harlow*

In the film *Dinner at Eight* (1933) Jean Harlow gives one of her finest comedic performances. Who can forget the sight of her lying in bed in a gorgeous negligee stuffing chocolates into her face?

"Venice is like eating an entire box of chocolate liqueurs in one go" —*Truman Capote*

truman capote

Legend has it that Albert Einstein was eating chocolate when he came upon the theory of relativity.

albert einstein

thomas jefferson

"The superiority of [hot] chocolate, both for health and nourishment, will soon give it the same preference over tea and coffee in America which it has in Spain"...

"Chocolate. ... By getting it good in quality, and cheap in price, the superiority of the article both for health and nourishment will soon give it the same preference over tea and coffee in America..."

—Thomas Jefferson, Paris, Nov. 27, 1785, to John Adams

"My secret passion has always been chocolate. Not just any chocolate. It has to be authentic chocolate. Chocolate as it has been prepared and consumed since the beginning of human history. There is nothing like sipping hot chocolate, sprinkled with cinnamon, as if I were a Maya Goddess. There is nothing like Mexican chocolate." —*Greta Garbo*

greta garbo

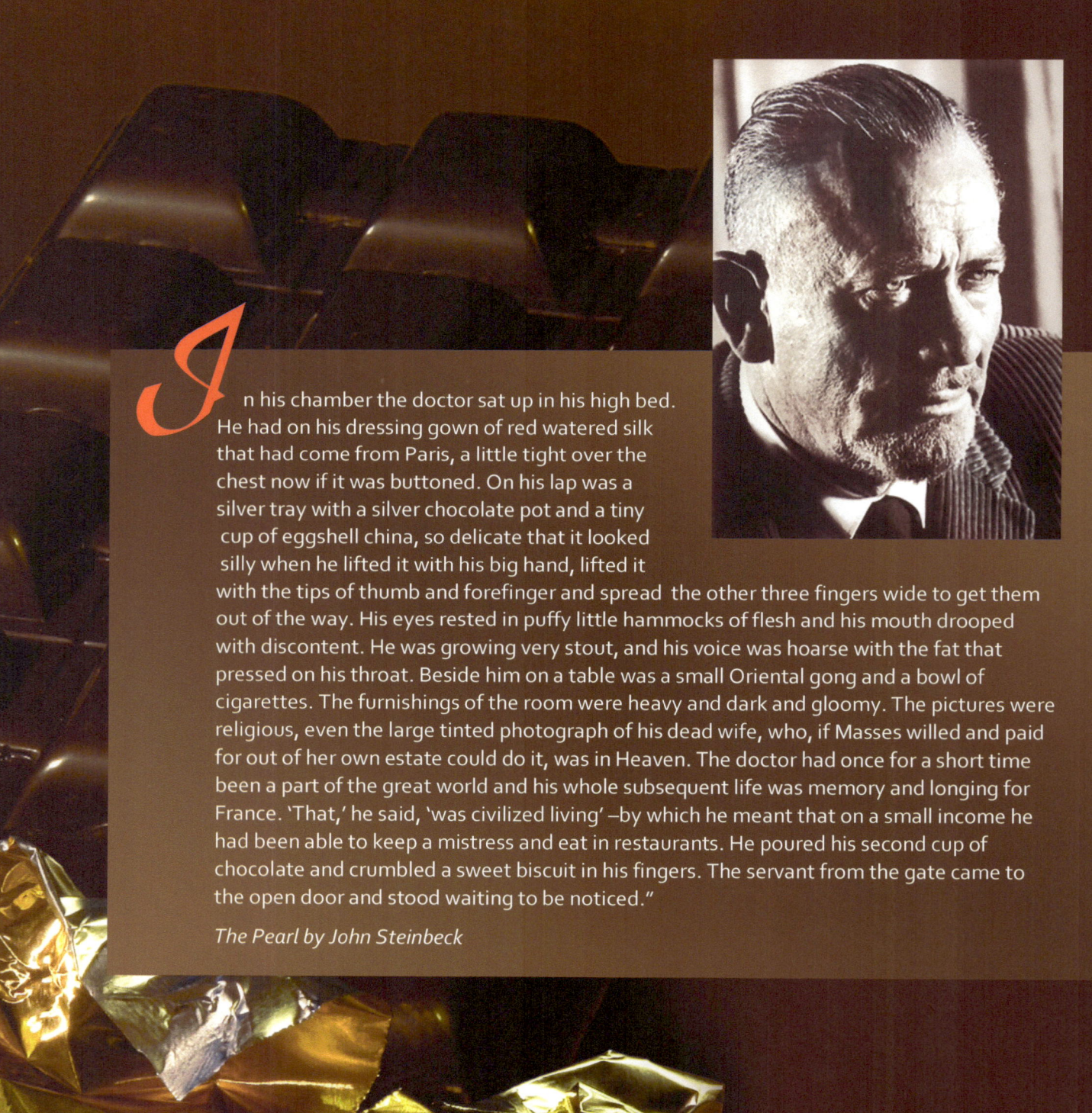

"In his chamber the doctor sat up in his high bed. He had on his dressing gown of red watered silk that had come from Paris, a little tight over the chest now if it was buttoned. On his lap was a silver tray with a silver chocolate pot and a tiny cup of eggshell china, so delicate that it looked silly when he lifted it with his big hand, lifted it with the tips of thumb and forefinger and spread the other three fingers wide to get them out of the way. His eyes rested in puffy little hammocks of flesh and his mouth drooped with discontent. He was growing very stout, and his voice was hoarse with the fat that pressed on his throat. Beside him on a table was a small Oriental gong and a bowl of cigarettes. The furnishings of the room were heavy and dark and gloomy. The pictures were religious, even the large tinted photograph of his dead wife, who, if Masses willed and paid for out of her own estate could do it, was in Heaven. The doctor had once for a short time been a part of the great world and his whole subsequent life was memory and longing for France. 'That,' he said, 'was civilized living' —by which he meant that on a small income he had been able to keep a mistress and eat in restaurants. He poured his second cup of chocolate and crumbled a sweet biscuit in his fingers. The servant from the gate came to the open door and stood waiting to be noticed."

The Pearl by John Steinbeck

glossary

Cacao: The tree from which chocolate is derived. Cacao trees grow in equatorial zones (20 degrees north and 20 degrees south of the equator) and produce large pods filled with seeds or beans. These are fermented and then processed to make various chocolate products.

Cocoa butter: The fat naturally present in cacao. It may be removed from roasted beans to separate it from cocoa powder. It can be added to chocolate to give it a richer mouth feel.

Cocoa liquor: A thick paste comprised of cocoa butter and cocoa solids, the result of grinding roasted and hulled cacao beans.

Cocoa mass: Cocoa liquor, but the term is used to refer to the combined percentage of all cocoa-based compounds in a chocolate bar compared with the proportion of sugar and other substances. Unsweetened chocolate is 100 percent cocoa mass and a moderately sweetened "bittersweet" bar will measure around 75 percent.

Cocoa nibs: The broken-up kernels of the cacao bean, usually extracted after fermentation, drying, and roasting of the beans and removal of the hulls is complete.

Conching: The grinding and refining process of the coarse and grainy cocoa mass along with additives, such as sugar and vanilla. Conching blends and aerates the ingredients over a few days into smooth chocolate, which can then be molded into bars.

Coverture: A high-quality chocolate with high cocoa butter content, ordinarily used as a coating for confections.

Criollo: The premium cacao variety. It has superior flavor and aroma. It is also the most difficult variety to cultivate.

Forastero: The second main variety of cacao, forastero is hardier and more abundant than criollo. It is, however, of lower quality than criollo, but it comprises the vast majority of world cacao production.

Ganache: A blend of chocolate, cream, and select (if any) flavoring ingredients, often used as a filling for truffles or fancy cakes.

Milk chocolate: The most common form of chocolate sold in the world. Milk solids are added to a combination of relatively high percentage of sugar and correspondingly lower percentage of cocoa solids.

Tempering: The process of cooling and reheating melted chocolate in a cyclical manner in order to create a stable crystalline structure producing a chocolate that's firm at room temperature, and has a distinct snap and gloss.

Trinitario: An eighteenth century criollo and forastero cacao hybrid. The idea was to produce cacao with the best characteristics of each of its progenitors for a wide market.

White chocolate: A combination of cocoa butter, vanilla, and sugar. It is not authentic chocolate because it lacks any cocoa solids.

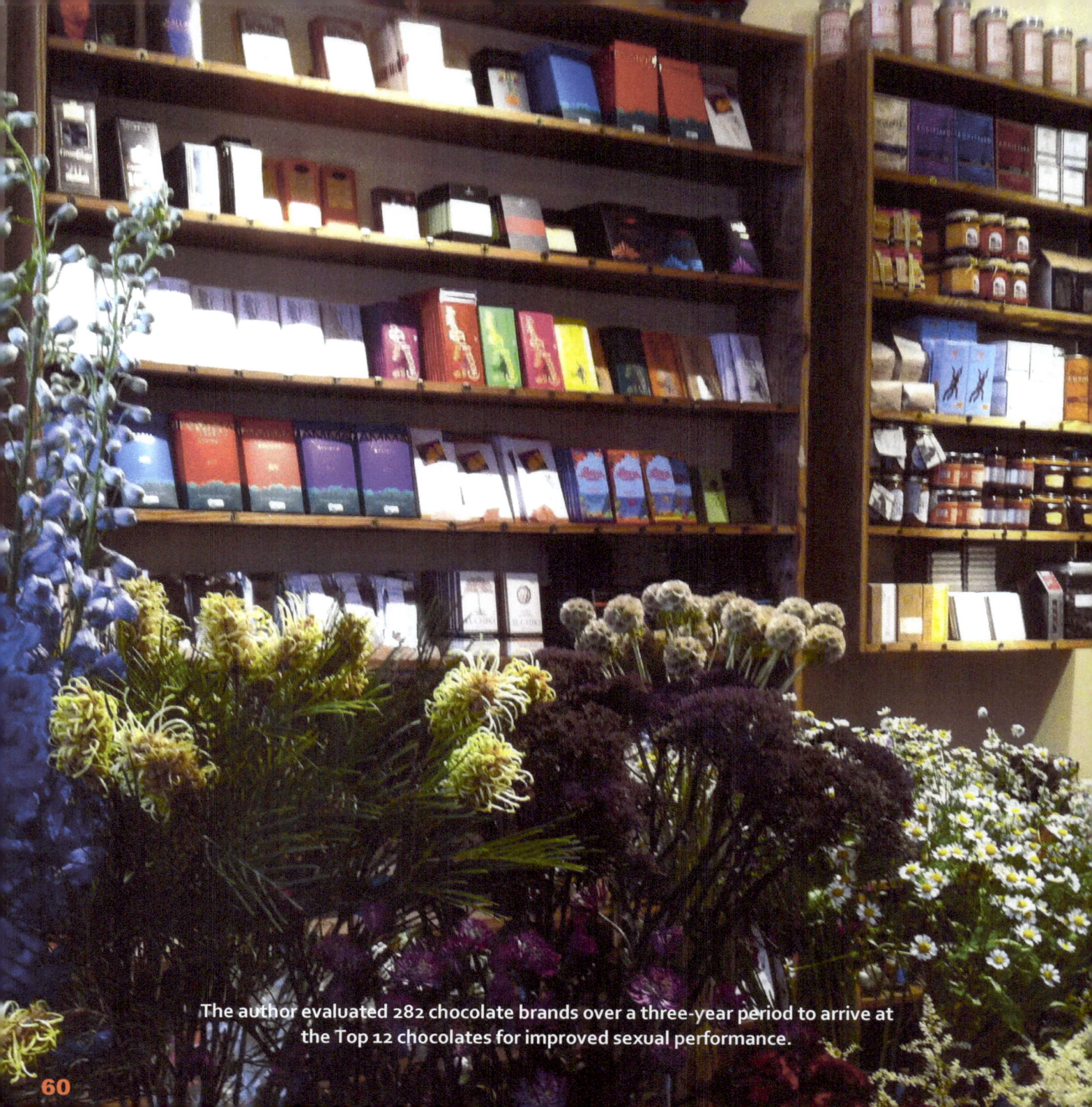

The author evaluated 282 chocolate brands over a three-year period to arrive at the Top 12 chocolates for improved sexual performance.

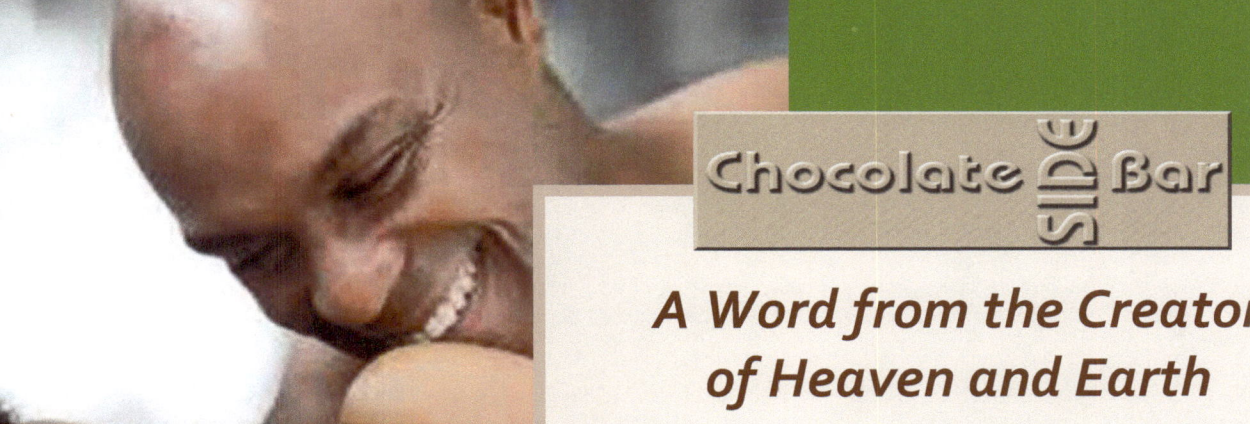

Chocolate SIDE Bar

A Word from the Creator of Heaven and Earth

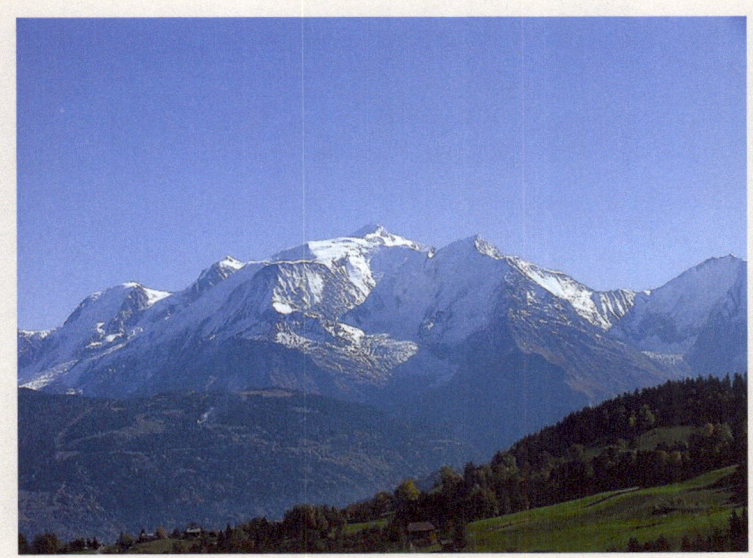

"Had I intended the Swiss to make chocolates, cacao trees would grow in the Alps." —*God*

notes

[1] See, *The True History of Chocolate* by Michael Coe, pages 28-29.

[2] "Effect of cocoa on blood pressure," by Ried K, Sullivan TR, Fakler P, Frank OR, Stocks NP; National Institute of IntegrativeMedicine, Melbourne, Australia.

[3] "Flavonoid-Rich Dark Chocolate Improves Endothelial Function and Increases Plasma Epicatechin Concentrations in Healthy Adults," by Engler MB, Engler MM, Chen CY, Malloy MJ, Browne A, Chiu EY, Kwak HK, Milbury P, Paul SM, Blumberg J, Mietus-Snyder ML, Laboratory of Cardiovascular Physiology, Department of Physiological Nursing, University of California, San Francisco, CA.

[4] "Effect of Dark Chocolate on Arterial Function in Healthy Individuals: Cocoa Instead of Ambrosia?" by Vlachopoulos C, Alexopoulos N, Stefanadis C., Hypertension Unit and Peripheral Vessels Unit, 1st Cardiology Department, Athens Medical School, Hippokration Hospital 17, Kerassoundos Str., Athens 11528, Greece.

[5] "Chocolate Consumption is Inversely Associated with Prevalent Coronary Heart Disease: The National Heart, Lung, and Blood Institute Family Heart Study," by Djoussé L, Hopkins PN, North KE, Pankow JS, Arnett DK, Ellison RC., Department of Medicine, Brigham and Women's Hospital and Harvard Medical School, Boston.

[6] "Blood Pressure and Cardiovascular Risk: What About Cocoa and Chocolate?" by Grassi D, Desideri G, Ferri C., Department of Internal Medicine and Public Health, University of L'Aquila, L'Aquila, Italy.

[7] "Effect of Dark Chocolate on Nitric Oxide Serum Levels and Blood Pressure in Prehypertension Subjects," by Sudarma V, Sukmaniah S, Siregar P., Departement of Clinical Nutrition, Faculty of Medicine, University of Indonesia, Jakarta Pusat, Indonesia.

[8] "Sexuality, Heart and Chocolate," by Bianchi-Demicheli F, Sekoranja L, Pechère-Bertschi A., Département de gynécologie et obstétrique, HUG, Genève, Switzerland.

[9] "Cocoa, Blood Pressure, and Vascular Function," by Sudano I, Flammer AJ, Roas S, Enseleit F, Ruschitzka F, Corti R, Noll G., Cardiovascular Center Cardiology, University Hospital Zurich, Raemistrasse 100, CH-8091, Zurich, Switzerland.

[10] "Chronic Consumption of Flavanol-Rich Cocoa Improves Endothelial Function and Decreases vascular Cell Adhesion Molecule in Hypercholesterolemic Postmenopausal Women," Wang-Polagruto JF, Villablanca AC, Polagruto JA, Lee L, Holt RR, Schrader HR, Ensunsa JL, Steinberg FM, Schmitz HH, Keen CL., Department of Nutrition, University of California, Davis, CA.

[11] "Effect of Consumption of Dark Chocolate on Oxidative Stress in Lipoproteins and Platelets in Women and in Men," Nanetti L, Raffaelli F, Tranquilli AL, Fiorini R, Mazzanti L, Vignini A., Department of Biochemistry, Biology and Genetics, Faculty of Medicine, Marche Polytechnic University, Via Tronto 10, Ancona, Italy.

[12] "The Impact of Chocolate on Cardiovascular Health," by Fernández-Murga L, Tarín JJ, García-Perez MA, Cano A., Fundación para la Investigación Hospital Universitario Dr Peset, Valencia, Spain.

[13] "Effect of Cocoa/Chocolate Ingestion on Brachial Artery Flow-Mediated Dilation and Its Relevance to Cardiovascular Health and Disease in Humans," by Monahan KD., Penn State Heart and Vascular Institute, Pennsylvania State University College of Medicine, Hershey, PA.

[14] See the section, "Slave-Tested, Master-Approved" for more information.

[15] See, Michael and Sophie Coe, *The True History of Chocolate*, page 57.

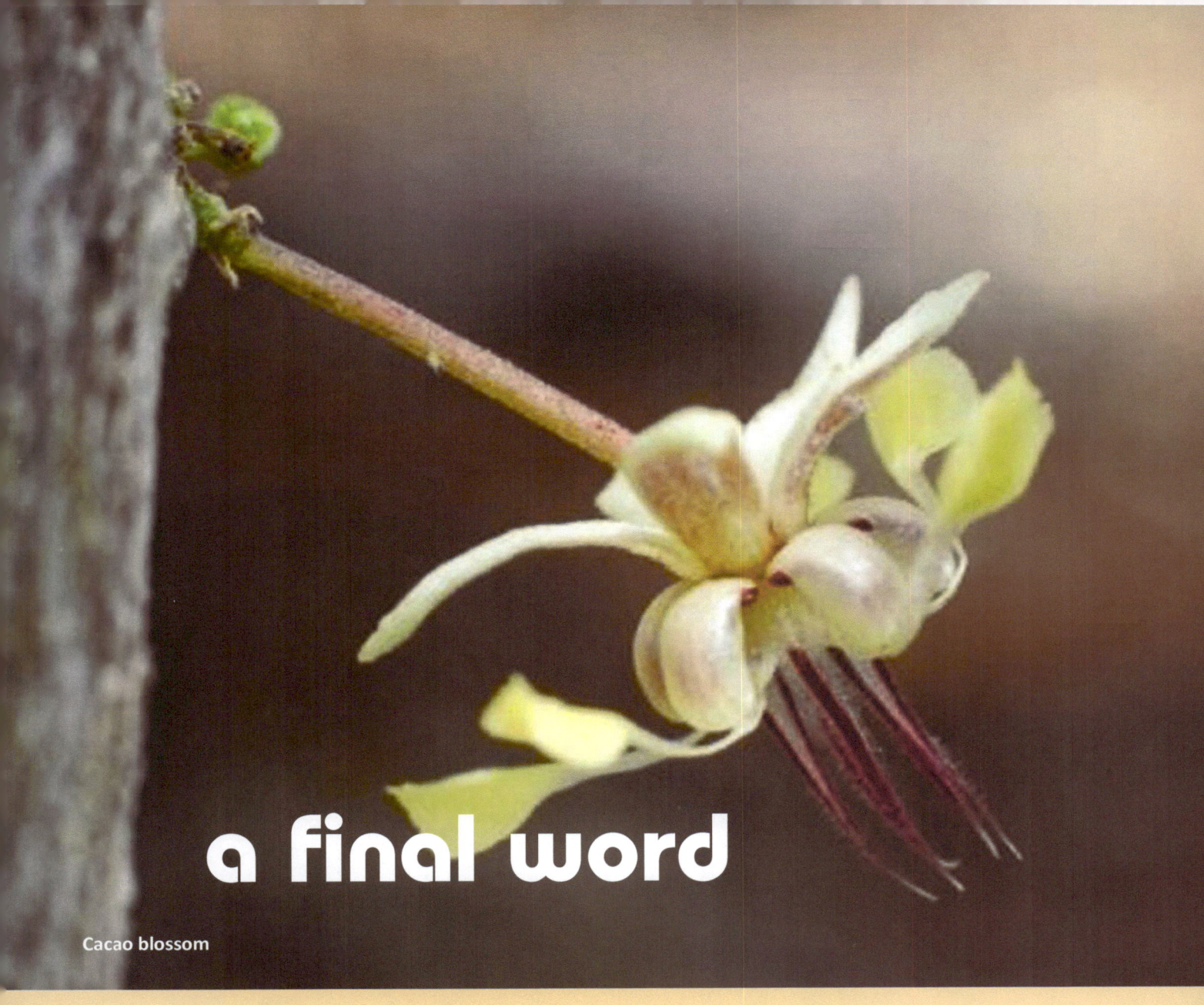

a final word

Cacao blossom

"I belong in the service of humanity"
— Song of the Mayab

www.ingramcontent.com/pod-product-compliance
Lightning Source LLC
Chambersburg PA
CBHW042029150426
43199CB00002B/15